Aphasia – A Social Approach

University

JOIN US ON THE INTERNET VIA WWW, GOPHER, FTP OR EMAIL:

WWW: http://www.thomson.com
GOPHER: gopher.thomson.com
FTP: ftp.thomson.com
EMAIL: findit@kiosk.thomson.com

A service of I(T)P

Aphasia – A Social Approach

Lesley Jordan
Middlesex University
Enfield
Middlesex
UK

and

Wendy Kaiser
Newcastle City Health Trust
Newcastle General Hospital
Newcastle upon Tyne
UK

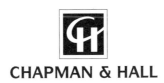

CHAPMAN & HALL
London · Weinheim · New York · Tokyo · Melbourne · Madras

Published by Chapman & Hall, 2–6 Boundary Row, London SE1 8HN, UK

Chapman & Hall, 2–6 Boundary Row, London SE1 8HN, UK

Chapman & Hall GmbH, Pappelallee 3, 69469 Weinheim, Germany

Chapman & Hall USA, 115 Fifth Avenue, New York NY 10003, USA

Chapman & Hall Japan, ITP-Japan, Kyowa Building, 3F, 2-2-1 Hirakawacho, Chiyoda-ku, Tokyo 102, Japan

Chapman & Hall Australia, 102 Dodds Street, South Melbourne, Victoria 3205, Australia

Chapman & Hall India, R. Seshadri, 32 Second Main Road, CIT East, Madras 600 035, India

Distributed in the USA and Canada by Singular Publishing Group Inc., 4284 41st Street, San Diego, California 92105

First edition 1996

© 1996 Lesley Jordan and Wendy Kaiser

Typeset in 10/12pt Times by Mews Photosetting, Beckenham, Kent

Printed in Great Britain by Alden Press, Osney Mead, Oxford

ISBN 0 412 49700 X   1 56593 197 1 (USA)

A catalogue record for this book is available from the British Library

Library of Congress Catalog Card Number: 96-85067

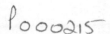

∞ Printed on permanent acid-free text paper, manufactured in accordance with ANSI/NISO Z39.48-1992 and ANSI/NISO Z39.48-1984 (Permanence of Paper).

Coventry University

To the memory of Diana Law
Founder and first President
of Action for Dysphasic Adults
A powerful aphasic communicator

Contents

Foreword

The social model of disability emerged from the work of the Union of the Physically Impaired Against Segregation (UPIAS) who published *The Fundamental Principles of Disability* in 1976. Central to this were two themes: that it was the experience and expertise of disabled people that was crucial in developing a true understanding of the phenomenon of disability and that the main problems of disabled people were externally located in the disabling barriers and social restrictions that they faced.

Building upon these themes and the rigid distinction between impairment and disability that the *Fundamental Principles* insisted upon, I further developed the social model as the basis of more appropriate professional practice as part of my own work in teaching disability issues to social workers (Oliver, 1983). Subsequently the social model became the accepted vehicle for the promotion and development of disability equality training (Campbell and Gillespie-Sells, 1991) and the basis of the collective self-organization of disabled people into a powerful political movement (Campbell and Oliver, 1996).

Outside of social work, the impact of the social model of disability on professional consciousness, let alone practice, has been somewhat limited. Medicine is still locked into the treatment and cure of impairments; physiotherapy and occupational therapy remain convinced that working in a one-to-one situation with disabled people on their functional limitations is the only way to proceed. Most of the rest of the professions still think that disabled people have something wrong with them and that individual therapy and compensation is the only appropriate approach to intervention.

It is thus refreshing to read a book that moves away from this position and takes the social model of disability as the vehicle for reflecting upon the practice of speech and language therapy for aphasic people. It begins quite properly with the experience of aphasia as an impairment before moving on to discuss current policies in respect of aphasia. The final section then uses the social model to discuss politics and power and their impact on the lives of aphasic people.

The book is not a professional textbook in the traditional sense of the term: it does not tell speech therapists how to implement the social model in working with disabled people. It recognizes that the social model implies a changed relationship between the professional and the disabled person requiring both a dialogue and a two-way sharing of expertise. It also explores methods of working with groups and other constituencies with a view to confronting and challenging externally imposed restrictions, from wherever they stem.

There is no doubt that the book makes an important contribution to the professional practice literature in that it reaches parts of the professional psyche not so far reached. It also raises the possibility that speech-impaired people can empower themselves through their own collective self-organization. If they do, then hopefully speech-impaired people will become much more centrally involved in the disability movement than they have been so far.

After all an empowered and powerful group of speech-impaired people are likely to make their collective voice heard throughout society, no matter what difficulties they have in speaking. If this book makes even a small contribution to this, then not only will professional practice become less disabling but we will all be living in a more inclusive society.

Mike Oliver
Professor of Disability Studies
University of Greenwich

REFERENCES

Campbell, J. and Gillespie-Sells, K. (1991) *A Guide to Disability Equality Training*, Central Council for the Education and Training of Social Workers, London.

Campbell, J. and Oliver, M. (1996) *Disability Politics: Understanding Our Past, Changing Our Future*, Routledge, London.

Oliver, M. (1983) *Social Work with Disabled People*, Macmillan, Basingstoke.

UPIAS (1976) *Fundamental Principles of Disability*, Union of the Physically Impaired Against Segregation, London.

Acknowledgements

Many people have contributed towards this book. First, there are the aphasic people and carers we interviewed and others who have written or recorded their accounts of life with aphasia. Next, we wish to thank a number of speech and language therapists and others involved in providing aphasia services. Rita Twiston Davies made a major contribution to the early thinking about the book. Jayne Cooper, Erica Crutchley, Maggie Fawcus, Roger Fitzsimmons, Stephanie Holland, Susie Parr, Carol Pound, Christina Shewell, Judith Williams and Carol Woods have given us help at various stages. Sally Byng's faith in our work has been an encouragement throughout. Staff at Action for Dysphasic Adults – Margaret Brandt, then Debby Rossiter and Ginni Tym, and more recently Ruth Coles and Lesley Axelrod – have answered numerous questions and provided much information. Likewise speech and language therapy managers, therapists and others providing services for aphasic people in the three districts studied in the late 1980s, and again in 1993, and speech and language therapy managers in the ten districts that responded to our request for information on pathways through aphasia services. Prue Oswin and Maree Miles have both been most helpful in ensuring that we were well informed about The Stroke Association services. Aura Kagan's inspirational work in Canada enabled us to follow through our exploration of the implications of the social model of disability. Comments on the manuscript made by Sally Byng and Barbara Waine have been enormously helpful. Maggie Boss gave invaluable help with proof-reading the book. Some of the research and writing was made possible by assistance from Middlesex University. We also owe a great deal to the forebearance and support of our families. The views stated in the book are those of the authors and are our responsibility alone.

Introduction

Communication – the imparting to another person or other people of information, ideas, thoughts and emotions – plays a central part in human life. The twentieth century has seen a technological transformation in our means of communication, especially via the telephone, radio, film, television and, increasingly, the Internet. Communication through the printed word has also expanded greatly. One thing that all these inventions have in common is their dependence, at least in part, on language as a means to convey messages. Language is important even where there is also a strong visual element. Silent movies, for example, used subtitles alongside other communication strategies including mime, gesture, body language and facial expression. Language is no less important as part of face-to-face interactions. We use it in many ways: to initiate, build and maintain relationships; to carry out transactions; to achieve status; to project our personalities; to assess other people. Language has been described as 'the core of what makes us human' (*The Mind Machine*, BBC2, 15 November 1988), and even as an instinct (Pinker, 1994).

Language comprises a number of different components, each of which requires a particular skill. It is often conceived mainly in terms of output, that is, speech and the written word. The parallel input skill for each mode, understanding speech and reading respectively, are equally essential for communication. Aphasia, the subject of this book, encompasses all language-related disorder resulting from damage to one or more of the brain's language centres. The term 'aphasia' derives from a Greek word meaning 'speechless', but the disorder may affect understanding of the spoken word, reading, writing, numerical skills and gesture, as well as speech itself. The combination of impairments and the specific nature and severity of each one vary widely from person to person. Barbara, a nurse who suffered a series of small strokes that caused temporary aphasia was able to describe how it had felt to be aphasic. She described having a 'pane of glass' inside her head that prevented words entering her mind. She could hear them but they 'slid off' the glass and she was unable to determine their meaning before the person spoke again. She felt similarly that the pane of glass prevented her from producing the words she wished to say. She was able to feel a response to a question building up in her head but was unable to get the words past the glass and thus out of her mouth.

As strokes are the commonest cause of aphasia, the book focuses on aphasia following stroke illness. What we say applies equally to the relatively small numbers of people who suffer from aphasia as a result of cerebral infections. The other significant causes of acquired aphasia are traumatic head injury and brain tumours. Whilst some aspects of the book will be relevant in relation to one or both of these groups, we do not attempt to cover the more complicated pattern of disability from head injury, nor the progressive nature of the condition in brain tumour. Although many people who suffer a stroke (though by no means all) are elderly, this book is concerned with adults of all ages who are aphasic following stroke.

The book is concerned with aphasia from three perspectives, which are analytically distinct but in practice inseparable. Our primary concern is with **people** affected by aphasia. First and foremost, this means aphasic people themselves. It also includes aphasic people's families and friends, whose lives may also be changed – at a stroke – by stroke. The consequences tend to be particularly marked for those who become carers.

The other set of people whose lives are influenced by aphasia are those who work to help aphasic people, either in a paid capacity or as volunteers. These people form a strong link to our second perspective, **policies**, since the framework for their work is set by the organizations that employ (or, in the case of volunteers, deploy) them. This framework will be mediated by various factors, including perceptions of aphasic people's needs, professional standards and wider policies, for example health service strategies at local and national levels. Our discussion in the book mainly concerns those people whose involvement is directly related to the aphasia. It is, however, important to note that other service providers may also be dealing with its effects. These might include, for example, doctors working in hospitals and in the community, physiotherapists, occupational therapists, social workers, benefits agency and employment services staff, clergy and others to whom aphasic people may turn.

An important aim of our twin focus on people and policies is to inform each about the other. Knowing about aphasic people's and their carers' wants, needs and preferences is essential if policies are to be sensitive and responsive to recipients. We concur with Anderson's conclusion (1992) to a longitudinal study of stroke that:

A sound, effective and ethical approach to stroke must lie in awareness of and attention to the experiences, values, priorities and expectations of patients and their carers – they are the people who live with the consequences of the illness and who shoulder its burdens.

(p. 217)

Equally, aphasic people and carers are likely to benefit from information about services, policies and the assumptions underlying them. Similarly, knowledge of the broader context within which they work should mean that front-line workers (including volunteers as well as professionals such as speech and language therapists), will be better able to protect and promote aphasic people's interests.

This brings us to our third, and in some ways least tangible perspective – **power**. Power means influence, authority and control over decisions. But we must look beyond the question of 'Who influenced this or that decision?' in order to understand where power lies. As Lukes (1974) argues, power may be exercised to prevent a particular decision being taken, or to define particular topics on to or off an agenda. Even more pervasive is influence over the shaping of people's wants and needs and of their perceptions of these. Another useful distinction is between 'power to' and 'power over' (p. 31). 'Power to' may mean the ability to achieve a desired end or to influence others. 'Power over' another person or group implies the ability to impose your will even against the wishes and/or interests of the other(s). Oliver (1990) discusses how professionals as a group wield power over disabled people, identifying a number of 'structures within which these power relations are located'. He continues:

> Economic structures determine the roles of professionals as gatekeepers of scarce resources, legal structures determine their controlling functions as administrators of services, career structures determine their decisions about whose side they are actually on and cognitive structures determine their practice with individual disabled people who need help – otherwise why would they be employed to help them?
>
> *(p. 90–1)*

The question at the end of this quotation implies that disabled people's need for help, in other words their dependence, is taken as given. At the individual level one person's increase in dependency upon another, perhaps for life's essentials, will mean a shift in the balance of power within that relationship. Further aspects of this power dimension will emerge as we consider the concept of disability.

DEFINING DISABILITY

The classification scheme of the World Health Organization (WHO) (1980) has been widely used. Its definitions of 'impairment', 'disability' and 'handicap' are shown in Table 1.1.

Table 1.1 The World Health Organization classification of disability

Impairment	Any loss or abnormality of psychological, physiological or anatomical structure or function
Disability	Any restriction or lack (resulting from an impairment) of ability to perform an activity in the manner or within the range considered normal for a human being
Handicap	A disadvantage for a given individual, resulting from an impairment or disability, that limits or prevents the fulfilment of a role (depending on age, sex, and social and cultural factors) for that individual

Source: WHO, 1980

This three-part definition of disability has several implications. We will consider these as they apply to aphasia. First, disability is a social construct, depending on judgements about the boundaries of 'normality'. This raises certain questions: How fixed are norms regarding language in a given culture? What assumptions are made about the language-disordered person? Can any negative assumptions be modified? If so, how and by whom? Second, disability can most usefully be conceived as a continuum, rather than as a discrete category (Martin *et al.*, 1988; Wood, 1989). Occasional word-finding problems and Spoonerisms, for example, are not seen as 'abnormal', or taken as evidence of underlying impairment. Such minor occurrences may be 'laughed off' or put down to fatigue, but might equally be understood as minimal aphasia. Third, aphasia is not a single disability, being more accurately described as a cluster of disabilities. For example, our list on p. 1 gives no fewer than six types of activity, or functions, that may be limited by aphasia. Fourth, brain damage that impairs language often at the same time causes other impairments. Many people aphasic as a result of stroke also have some degree of impairment of walking, dexterity and/or sight. Anderson found that speech-impaired people made 'less physical recovery' and were more likely than others to remain severely disabled 18 months after their stroke (1992).

Finally, the WHO's conceptualization of 'handicap' means that the impact of similar disability may differ among individuals. Being unable to make sense of the written word, for example, will be a major problem for someone who was formerly an avid reader, but may have less significance for a person who read very little before becoming aphasic. Handicap depends on each individual's circumstances, including the person's own reaction to becoming and being disabled in particular ways, the roles previously held, factors in the environment that enable or preclude continuance of these roles and/or development of new ones, and other people's reactions and their assumptions about appropriate roles for the disabled person and for themselves in relation to that person. Safilios-Rothschild suggests in relation to this last point that: 'the disabled person is often considered to be less intelligent, less able to make the 'right' decisions, less 'realistic', less logical, and less able to determine his own life than a non-disabled person' (1981, p. 5). Disabled people's self-images will be affected by other people's behaviour towards them and vice versa (Block and Yuker, 1979). The WHO categorization is used in a number of countries (Worrall, 1992; Holland, 1993) 'as cardinal to notions of functionalism in treatment for aphasia' (Holland, 1993, x).

The WHO classification has been criticized by the disability movement in Britain on many counts, including its tendency to individualize and pathologize all problems associated with disability and its negative stereotyping of disabled people. Disabled writers have labelled such models 'personal tragedy' (Oliver, 1983, 1990) or 'social death' models (Finkelstein, 1991, after Miller and Gwynne, 1972). Their alternative, the social model, is based on the observation that disabled people are disadvantaged by the way our society is structured. The social model of disability is sometimes called the 'social barriers' (Finkelstein) or 'social oppression' (Oliver) model. Its definitions are shown in Table 1.2.

Table 1.2 Social model definition of disability

Impairment	The functional limitation within the individual caused by the lack of part or all of a limb, or having a defective limb, organ, or physical, mental or sensory mechanism of the body[a]
Disability	The loss or limitation of opportunities that prevents people who have impairments from taking part in the normal life of the community on an equal level with others owing to physical and social barriers[b]

Sources: [a]This definition of impairment combines those of Barnes (1991), and Finkelstein and French (1993).
[b]Finkelstein and French (1993).

The social model definition of 'impairment' is compatible with the WHO schema. This definition encompasses the functional aspect of disability as presented by the WHO. The distinguishing feature of the disability movement's approach lies in its definition of 'disability', with its emphasis on the disabling effects of factors external to the individual, and hence its implied agenda for societal change. The movement's demands include rights of access to services and a new relationship with those who provide them, a more accessible environment and anti-discrimination legislation (Finkelstein, 1993). The disability movement also rejects the term 'handicap' (Barnes, 1991). Table 1.3 provides a comparison of the individual and social model approaches to disability.

Concern is being expressed within the disability movement that the need to present a positive image of disabled people in order to counteract long-established negative views has sometimes led to a denial of the personal experience of disablement (Morris, 1991; French, 1993a). As Morris states: 'Disability *is* associated with illness, and with old age ... and with conditions which are inevitably painful' (1991, p. 181, italics original). There is no doubt that people who become aphasic commonly experience their impairment as a severe loss, at least initially (see Chapter 2). Also, disabled people often require particular services because of their impairment, a point perhaps not fully acknowledged within the social model (French, 1993a).

Table 1.3 Comparison of models of disability

Model of disability	Individual model	Social model
Other labels	Personal tragedy model Individual pathology model Social death model Medical model	Social barriers model Social oppression model
Orientation to disability	Disability *per se* seen as a problem	Disability seen as part of life; not necessarily problematic
Main source of problems disabled people encounter	Individual disabled person's impairment	Society's failure to meet needs of all its members
Primary focus	Diversity of disabling conditions – disabled people as separate individuals	Problems/interests in common – disabled people as a group
Orientation to disabled people's lives	Disabled life devalued as 'not worth living'	Disabled people and their contribution to life valued
Activity orientation	Functional limitations: 'things disabled people can't do'	People's abilities: we all have abilities – and things we can't do
Policy orientation	Administrative 'solutions'	Civil rights/equal opportunities
Type of service preferred	Segregated provisions as most efficient way to deal with/hide the problem	Integrated provision to enable disabled people to participate in full in society
Main focus of health/rehabilitation services	Treat impairment; improve person's level of functioning	Remove social barriers: increase people's control over their lives
Power to determine services disabled people require	Health and welfare professionals and officials, on assessments of need	Disabled people, based on their perceptions of need and calling on professionals as a resource

The assumptions underlying the individual pathology model are deeply imbedded in our culture. Disabled people will encounter them frequently. Many disabled people's (and their significant others') perceptions of their own experience of disability are undoubtedly shaped by these assumptions. Finkelstein (1991) suggests that a system to administer services to disabled people is the corollary of a social death model and also that 'administrative approaches dominate all forms of helping services for disabled people in the UK, whether these are provided by statutory agencies or voluntary charities, or demanded by pressure-group organisations' (Finkelstein, 1993, p. 37). As suggested above, the individual model of disability leads to the social construction of dependency for disabled people, both as a group and individually (Oliver, 1990). It thus places disabled people in a position of powerlessness. The social model is important because it sees disability as an equal opportunities issue. This insight is a prerequisite for the empower-ment of disabled people, as well as having far-reaching implications for policy and practice. We explore some of these as they apply to aphasia in later chapters.

We have found it necessary to draw on both individual and social mod-els of disability. Focusing only on the type of impairment inevitably runs the risk of neglecting the person as a whole. We are only too aware of this danger. We have attempted to avoid slipping into a condescending 'per-sonal tragedy' mode of thinking ourselves, whilst recognizing disabled people's right to feel and express their sense of shock and distress. With few exceptions, aphasia services are grounded in the individual pathology model. In order to understand these services in their own terms, we make use of the individual pathology framework and definitions. We do, how-ever, attempt throughout to move beyond this model, in order to discuss the implications for aphasia therapy and other aphasia services of the social model.

A NOTE ON TERMINOLOGY

We need to clarify our use of the terms aphasia and dysphasia. **Aphasia** means, literally, a complete absence of speech. In Britain, the more accurate term **dysphasia** (lack of coordination in speech/difficulties with speech) has commonly been used in relation to all but the most severely afflicted. Following North American and European usage, however, there is a grow-ing preference in Britain for the term 'aphasia'. We comply with this trend, using 'dysphasia' only in quotations and proper names. The reader should treat the two words as interchangeable.

Aphasic people are referred to as, for example, **patients** within the National Health Service (NHS), **clients** of a Communication Aid Centre, and **students** in the context of adult basic education services. Where we are presenting material that relates to a particular service we use its terminology. Except when referring to published accounts, videos or audiocassettes, we have changed names of aphasic people and carers to protect their anonymity.

In Britain, the profession most involved with aphasic people has been called **speech and language therapy** since 1991. Between 1945 and 1991 the profession was called speech therapy so this term appears in our text where we quote from pre-1991 documents. In much of Europe the equivalent professionals are called logopaedists or orthophonistes, in the USA speech pathologists and in Canada speech–language pathologists. Unless otherwise specified, the terms **therapist**, **clinician** and **clinical supervisor** refer to speech and language therapists in this book. Speech and language therapists who specialize in treating aphasic people may be termed **aphasia therapists** and those who study aphasia **aphasiologists**.

PLAN OF THE BOOK

The book is in three parts. Part One is concerned mainly with aphasic people and the meaning of aphasia to them. In Chapter 2 we attempt to understand how people experience aphasia and the economic and social implications of being aphasic in our society. Chapter 3 discusses the nature of the communication disorder and how it occurs, and summarizes some information on incidence and prevalence. Part Two is about services that aim to help aphasic people with communication and the policies on which they are based. In Chapter 4 we explore aphasia therapy and look at evaluation of its outcome. Chapter 5 examines the pattern of aphasia services for populations and individuals in Britain, and Chapter 6 locates these services in a wider context. Chapter 7 considers volunteer involvement. In Part Three we draw the three themes of people, policies and power together, aiming to provide a blueprint for a social model approach to aphasia, using some recent initiatives by way of illustration. Chapter 8 focuses on the implications of the social model for aphasia therapy. Chapter 9 is much broader in scope; in this concluding chapter we follow through the application of social model ideas for many aspects of aphasic people's lives.

A GUIDE FOR READERS

We have aimed to write a book that is usable and useful as well as being readable. We have tried to keep the book free of jargon; where the use of technical terms has been unavoidable we have taken care to explain them in lay language. Different groups of readers might choose to approach the book in different ways. We anticipate that those new to aphasia and wanting an introduction to the whole area, such as students, will start at the beginning and read through to the end. Readers whose primary interest is in the lived experience of aphasia should turn first to Chapters 2 and 9. Aphasic people and carers will find Chapters 3 and 4 useful in explaining the disorder and aphasia therapy, but may judge the detailed discussion of service provision in Chapters 5 and 6 less relevant to them. In providing an overview of what it is like to be aphasic, or to live with someone who is aphasic, Chapter 2 will be very relevant to all concerned with helping aphasic people. Chapters 4 and 8 may be of most interest to speech and language therapists and others who wish to understand the work they do, since these chapters focus on aphasia therapy *per se*. Chapter 7 is also much concerned with speech and language therapists' roles, but this time specifically in relation to volunteers. It will be of relevance to all those involved with volunteering, whether volunteers themselves, organizers or managers. Chapters 5 and 6 should be of particular interest to those responsible for managing aphasia services, either as purchasers or providers. Whilst they might decide to miss out Chapters 3 and 4, the final section of each of these chapters addresses management issues. Chapter 3 may be read in detail by readers who want to acquire some physiological or neurological understanding of aphasia, and will no doubt be avoided by others. Short sections on topics such as residential care and employment are included in several chapters, so these themes could be followed through quite easily. Another recurring theme, addressed particularly in Chapters 2, 4, 5, 6, 8 and 9, concerns carers' roles.

Readers concerned with aphasia in countries other than the UK should not be discouraged by the fact that *Aphasia – A Social Approach* is based primarily on British evidence and experience. Many of the issues discussed in the book are not peculiar to the UK and we draw on material from a range of other countries wherever possible. The organization and financing of health and social care do, of course, vary considerably from country to country. Chapters 5 and 6 make no attempt to go beyond analysis of the British system. Our examination of provision in Britain should, however, enable readers with knowledge of services elsewhere to make comparisons.

This book is the first attempt, as far as we know, to consider the implications of the social model of disability in such detail in relation to a particular impairment. Readers approaching it as a social model case study may wish to concentrate on Chapter 2, the sections on social model practice in Chapters 4 and 7, and Part Three.

If you have started reading at the 'Plan of the Book' section (a ploy we tend to use ourselves!), we recommend that you now read the rest of the Introduction. This explains our approach to the individual and social models of disability that provide the book's theoretical underpinning, and aims to clarify the book's rationale.

PART ONE

People

Living with aphasia

An understanding of how aphasia has affected other people's lives may be supportive to aphasic people and their carers. It is also important in order to foster personal interactions, services and policies that are sensitive to aphasic people's and carers' needs. In this chapter we look at aphasia mainly through the eyes of people who have written or talked about their experience of it. We use quotations and case histories drawn from a number of sources, including published and unpublished written accounts, videos and audiocassettes, discussion with speech and language therapists, and a small number of interviews with aphasic people and close relatives.

As has been stated in Chapter 1, aphasia is a very variable condition. The specific ways it impairs language will differ markedly from person to person and may change for one person during the course of the day as well as over the months and years. Reliance as far as possible on aphasic people's own accounts inevitably introduces a bias towards those who have made a relatively good recovery in terms of communication. The nature and severity of the impairment by no means determines people's experience of disablement. Bury (1991) alerts us to the importance of taking into account 'the positive actions people adopt to counter the effects of symptoms and treatment' (p. 460). Responses to becoming and being aphasic also vary. We would expect responses to be mediated by the individual's life experiences (based in a particular culture, class and gender) and personality, and to be ongoing and to change over time. Bury identifies three dimensions of people's reactions to chronic illness (equally applicable to impairment following stroke) that he calls 'coping', 'strategy' and 'style'. **Coping** concerns the construction people put on their impairment and the attitudes they hold or develop in relation to living with it; Bury suggests that successful coping 'involves maintaining a sense of value and meaning in life, in spite of symptoms and their effects'.

Strategy means 'the actions people take, or *what people do* in the face of illness' and, more specifically, 'the actions taken to mobilise resources and maximise favourable outcomes'. **Style** 'refers to *the way* people respond to, and present, important features of their illness or treatment regimes' (pp. 461–2, italics original). For people whose preferred style is to verbalize what has happened to them, becoming aphasic may be particularly disruptive.

Our aim in this chapter is to illustrate some of the effects of aphasia and people's ways of dealing with it, in order to provide qualitative insights into aphasic living. We start by focusing on communication itself, before discussing aphasic people's feelings about their impairment and themselves. Then we consider in turn how various aspects of an individual's life may be affected and examine the impact of aphasia on family life. We view the aphasic person throughout not merely as a passive receptacle of the disorder and recipient of services but as 'someone who plays an active role in the process of developing a new, constructive, potent disabled identity' (Parr, Pound and Marshall, 1995, p. 9). We conclude by discussing recent research that draws a number of these strands together.

COMMUNICATION

Since (as was noted in the Introduction) so many human activities involve some form of language, aphasia is an extremely pervasive disability. Some aphasic people are unable to make sense of the written word, and therefore cannot read books, newspapers or letters. Many aphasic people find watching television very tiring, so can view for only short periods. Television and radio programmes may be only partially understood or completely incomprehensible, reducing the pleasure they give or making viewing or listening impossible. Activities such as travel, shopping and using the phone are likely to be affected. Communication is the medium through which human associations are made and maintained, so an aphasic person's family, social and other relationships may suffer. In general, aphasia can have the effect of cutting people off from many aspects of life. Our contention that this is not inevitable is explored in later chapters.

Table 2.1 summarizes the communication difficulties reported by informal 'supporters' of a sample of stroke patients in the London Borough of Greenwich (Anderson, 1992). Nearly half the supporters recorded that the stroke patient had difficulties in 'speaking what he/she wants to say', although only 32% of the patients were formally assessed as having such impairments. Self-reported difficulties came between these figures, with 42% of the patients themselves describing 'a problem finding words' (p. 167). Visual and physical impairments will account for a proportion of these communication problems. The relationship between language impairment and memory is uncertain. Hearing difficulties are included here for comparison.

Table 2.1 Supporters' assessments of difficulties patients had with communication 18 months after stroke

Patient had difficulty:	Proportion of supporters who felt the patient had difficulty
Hearing a normal conversation	36% (75)[a]
Understanding a normal conversation	35% (75)
Speaking what he/she wanted to say	48% (75)
Reading	47% (70)
Writing	69% (75)
Remembering things	50% (76)

[a]Figures in brackets are the numbers on which the percentages are based.
Source: Anderson (1992) Table 59, p. 168.

Slack's perceptive account (Slack and Mulville, 1988) of caring for Adeline, her elderly, aphasic mother, illustrates clearly a mosaic of communication abilities alongside the language impairment. Despite a complete absence of speech following a major stroke, Adeline gradually regained the ability to make herself understood, using gesture, facial expression and intonation. 'No-one could have been in any doubt as to whether lo, la, lo, la, lo was said approvingly, disapprovingly, in horror, in amazement, to ask a question or to acquiesce' (p. 103). Adeline could not identify an object such as a cup out of context but, when asked, could set the table using the correct number of cups and saucers. If taken to the supermarket, she could select her preferred brands of common foods. She could also recognize familiar handwriting.

Ireland (Ireland and Black, 1992) also makes the distinction between language and communication:

I have a language problem, not a communication problem. Part of brain is dead but with a loss also a gain if work to build inner insight and strength. I think I am better communicator than before the stroke. ... I can't flannel now. My language is closer to my feelings. But it could be more difficult people to hear it cause people need flannel particularly to receive a critical issue, something challenging.

(p. 355)

We now examine further the effects of aphasia in relation to spoken and written communication.

Conversation

Anderson's research findings confirm that aphasia is associated with a reduction in conversation. Half the supporters of speech-impaired patients reported that 'the patient conversed much less than before the stroke ... compared with 15% of other supporters' (1992, p. 168).

From our own research, Ken encapsulates the close relationship between thought and language: 'Not just the words themselves are missing, but the whole idea of seeking to clothe ideas in words.' At a more practical level, Charles describes his problems: 'After my stroke I could only answer questions by nodding and shaking my head. Sometimes I was able to say yes or no.' Julia could say only one word when she first came out of her coma. This was 'on'. It was about a month before her speech began to recover. Three years on: 'my words come out the wrong way'. Julia also has difficulty if her train of thought is interrupted. If someone butts in, she mixes up what she wants to say with what she has already said. Ben found that:

> Everything is too fast. People talk to you at a normal speed and you remember only the last few words of what they are saying. This is frustrating when you have something to add to a conversation and they haven't time to hear what you have to say.

In contrast, Logan (1994) writes: 'I could understand everything clearly, and at speed. One of the most condescending things, was for people to talk to you as if you were 'thick'. Aphasic people complain of being spoken to in baby language and of people shouting at them. Jim (Action for Dysphasic Adults (ADA) audiocassette *Living with Dysphasia*, 1993) describes how friends reacted by ignoring his wife:

> Initially, as people realised that Dorothy couldn't take part in the conversation, they would talk to me. Perhaps Dorothy would be sat between two of us and they would talk about her, and over her, and through her, to me. And Dorothy would be sat, as though she was attending a tennis match, looking from one to the other, but nobody was really talking to her. And that was extremely frustrating, and as far as Dorothy was concerned, it made her very angry. I would say occasionally 'Dorothy understands. Will you talk to her please.' ... This has developed over the years so that people do talk to Dorothy and understand that she knows what's going on.

Casual acquaintances may assume that the aphasic person's silence signifies unwillingness to speak. Elsie relates a hospital porter's words to her: 'When you first came to [hospital] you were a poor little thing. You sat in the corner and wouldn't talk to anyone.'

Speech difficulties can render a person socially impotent. Note the porter's description of Elsie as a 'poor little thing'. We know several instances of aphasic people longing to tell jokes again, but afraid to try because they cannot be sure of being able to deliver the punch line. Some non-aphasic people try to help out by supplying what they guess is the word or phrase that an aphasic person is struggling to produce. This may work if the conversation partner is in tune with the aphasic person's thoughts and ideas, and some aphasic people find it acceptable. Others prefer to be given the time they need to convey their own message. On the ADA audiocassette *Personal Insights* (1995) aphasic people describe how annoying they find such behaviour and how it may lead to misunderstandings. Frank noticed that after his stroke some acquaintances would cross over the street to avoid having to acknowledge him.

Ken's experience was somewhat different. He wrote: 'As kind as people are, they "damn me with faint praise", make "allowances for me" and listen to my conversation with "kindly understanding". There are exceptions to this, of course.' As implied here, by no means all the experiences we heard about were negative. Julia, travelling home on her own from her new day centre, found herself on the wrong train. The young man sitting opposite her backed away initially on hearing that Julia had had a stroke, but then changed his mind and even waited with her for another train at the terminus.

Strategies adopted to replace or aid speech varied widely, both in nature and in acceptability to other people. In the ADA video Say the words that matter, Graham relates how he attracted the nurses' attention in hospital by throwing things at their office, as he was unable to call them. The nurses thought he was delirious. Some people find it helpful to write the first letter of what they want to say on paper or in the air, while others write whole messages. Holland (1982) describes other strategies, such as finding an object, and using mime, gesture and humour.

Many severely aphasic people are unable to use the telephone at all. Our impression is that, for those who can, a distinction needs to be made between different kinds of calls. Several of the people we spoke to were able to make and/or take social calls, but could not manage more formal calls, for example to obtain information or discuss business matters.

Communication in a group often poses considerable problems. It is difficult for someone with aphasia to keep track of several different threads of conversation, especially if there is more than one person speaking at once, and/or background noise. Group communication tends to be more disjointed than one-to-one and this, plus the effort of listening to or understanding several different communicative styles, may tire the aphasic person. Fatigue affects comprehension and so it is harder to attend to what is being said. The strategy that scriptwriter Leon Griffiths adopted if a group discussion went too fast for him to follow was to sit back and look wise (Chest, Heart and Stroke Association, (CHSA) video *Back to Square One*). Avoidance of social activities that involved more than a few people was another strategy, but one that had a limiting effect on people's lives, ruling out parties, going to public houses and many other activities.

Reading and writing

The use of literacy skills varies considerably from person to person depending on their roles in various spheres of life – domestic, work, leisure, etc. This is clearly illustrated by Parr's research (1995). To explore factors affecting aphasic people's linguistic practices and needs she interviewed 20 aphasic people, where possible with their partners. Parr identified no fewer than 23 specific reading or writing tasks that aphasic people wanted to be able to do again, and 'no two subjects cited the same combination of activities' (p. 230). Reading tasks mentioned included looking up information and following instructions of various kinds as well as reading books and newspapers. Specific examples were: using a phone directory, reading instructions on food packets and cans and reading children's stories aloud. Some of the writing tasks identified included those for everyday business, such as writing cheques or a shopping list; others had more to do with leisure or social activities, like filling in a betting slip or writing postcards.

One of the best-known accounts of living with aphasia, that by Ritchie (1960, 1974) grew out of a diary that the author began to write at the suggestion of a speech therapy student as part of his therapy. He records: 'It began with blank pages and much mental pain. After a bit I allowed words to creep in on me, words that meant nothing; then I found myself recording how I felt and how life went at the [rehabilitation] Centre' (1974, p. 115). Alan was able to copy writing accurately, but not to construct a sentence. He wrote to his sister, but made 'so many mistakes'. He sometimes knew he had made a mistake but could not correct it himself.

Ireland (Ireland and Black, 1992) describes graphically her difficulties in writing:

> I have feeling that I want to write. So difficult the mechanics re writing: translate thoughts to words, put together with grammar, forgetting the right spellings, haltering to express the right climate. Haltering words and hearing out aloud to write down – then I forgot the thought!
>
> *(p. 358)*

Some of Parr's interviewees gave 'evidence of adaptation to aphasia through the use of social, operational and technical back-ups' (1995, p. 233). Social back-up here means obtaining help from another person whilst retaining some responsibility for the task, and thereby at least partially maintaining a particular role. Operational back-up might involve the development of drafting, editing and proof-reading techniques. Technical aids used by Parr's interviewees (1995) included 'depending on television and radio to supplement news intake from papers, memory buttons on phones and the use of credit cards and cash dispensers to circumvent cheque-writing' (p. 232). Other technical aids might include talking books and computers, a word processor having the advantage of enabling aphasic people themselves to correct their written output easily and reliably. Margot received a bursary from the British Aphasiology Society for a word-processing course (ADA *Personal Insights* audiocassette, 1995).

HOW IT FEELS TO BE APHASIC

A number of factors will affect how disabled an aphasic person feels. The severity of the speech and language disability may be less significant than the person's ability to communicate and the importance of language and communication in her or his life. Initial reactions range from laughter to feeling utterly mystified. Where aphasia is the only symptom of a stroke, bewilderment has on occasion been increased by misdiagnosis of a psychiatric condition. Some aphasic people have described their initial certainty that their language would return to normal soon, and as suddenly as it had gone.

From published accounts by people who have become aphasic, Lebrun (1978) identifies alternative initial responses of fear and indifference. The former is easily understandable; the latter may stem from an 'upsetting of the intellectual faculties [which] prevents the patient from realizing the full scope of his impairment' (p. 51). Many people can remember little about the early days of their illness. As Elsie wrote:

> The first thing I knew about being ill was listening to my husband on the telephone and being taken backwards and forwards to [the hospital] for speech therapy. Thinking about this I feel as though part of my life is missing.
>
> *(Unpublished account written for Speak Week, 1987)*

Others retain their awareness, as in the following account, which also describes the writer's feelings during the ensuing weeks:

> I awoke about 3 a.m. and I sensed there was something wrong. My head was clear enough but I realised that I was completely paralysed down my right side and I couldn't utter a sound ... Through the weeks that followed my main worry was my inability to speak which was terribly hard to bear ... Eventually, I managed to string 'good morning' and 'good evening' together and this did wonders for my morale ... The effects of intensive physiotherapy and my body getting stronger seemed to trigger off a gradual recovery of my speech, also the assessment of my speech therapist that I would continue to improve, cheered me up no end ... I feel that whatever form of disability the stroke patient has to come to terms with, the loss of speech

due to the frustration and anxiety it imposes on that person, must put it very high on any list.

(ADA, 1982)

In the early days and weeks, feelings of helplessness and confusion are common. Being severely aphasic may mean being unable to communicate even your most basic needs. For this reason stroke patients are sometimes wrongly diagnosed as incontinent (e.g. Campling, 1981). Malcolm says of the time just after he came out of hospital: 'I was in a daze. I can't do it anything properly.' For George: 'At first speech was very difficult. I could speak very little – just "yes" and "no".' He was confused mainly because he couldn't understand what people were saying: 'I thought I could understand, but obviously I couldn't.' Alan remembers feeling very tired and weak when he first returned home from hospital after his stroke. For about 6 months people found his speech unintelligible. He says of that time: 'It's emotional that I can't speak. I was unhappy 'cause I can't speak.'

It has been suggested that many people go through a period of complete misery as comprehension and awareness of their problems improve. Währborg discusses this reactive state, as well as possible organic (biochemical) causes of depression (1991; see also Chapter 3). Malcolm describes his feelings: 'I am impatient with myself because I can't talk properly. Frustrating ... apart from my business [which he had to sell] I feel very miserable sometimes because I can't make people understand me so I can't say to you how I feel ... sometimes, I could weep.' He summed up the effect on his life in one word: 'catastrical'.

Another emotion that arises is anger. Ireland (Ireland and Black, 1992) expresses this evocatively, showing also her sense of loss:

> Everyday is not a joy. Daily demands. Travelling difficult, noise and nausea. I can very aware of the noise. External noise interview ... interferes me to listen. I can't concentrate with it. I can't screen it out. I so want to be involved with life, which I did before, but there is a little bit of me which is still difficult accepting my limits. Pain permanetes in my life. Try pain-killers, acupuncture, massage, yoga, relaxation. Often anger about it. I will to live active and enjoyable life. So hard to find out better how to do it.

(p. 356)

This passage illustrates clearly how the whole experience of disabling factors contributes to the struggle of day-to-day living with impairment.

As well as leading to feelings of confusion, misery, anger, loss and intense frustration, being aphasic can be a very isolating experience. The majority of the speech-impaired stroke patients in Anderson's study (1992) said they felt lonely, compared with a quarter of non-speech-impaired stroke patients. Feelings of aloneness can occur even when communication is relatively good. This may be because non-aphasic people do not share the experience of disability, and many are unwilling or unable to allow the aphasic person to express feelings, concerns and fears that they cannot share and do not understand. Where such feelings are expressed, they may be discounted or receive a negative response. This is illustrated by the following case study.

> Julia's stroke occurred when she was 17 and followed an operation. Despite being in a coma for 2 weeks, she made a good recovery, and 3 years later had little difficulty in making herself understood, though she was still noticeably aphasic. She had recently started to become very nervous of going to bed for fear of suffering another stroke and dying in bed. This fear may have been triggered by a pain that her doctor diagnosed as indigestion. He also prescribed sleeping pills. Julia felt that her doctor didn't understand her. She couldn't talk to her mother: 'When I say something, have a conversation, she backs away. She treats me like a child.' She felt the one friend she could confide in 'is sick of it' and that it would be embarrassing to talk to other people about her fears.

Julia experienced her doctor's concentration on her physical symptoms as a denial of her quite natural worries about her health. Her mother's reaction fits in closely with the stereotype of the disabled identified by Safilios-Rothschild (1981) and quoted in Chapter 1.

Another feeling common to many disabled people is of stigma, of being 'disqualified from full social acceptance' (Goffman, 1968, p. 9). Stigma originates partly in the attitudes and actions of others, which may restrict the options for the disabled person. People with communication impairment may be particularly vulnerable to having people talking about them in their presence as if they weren't there, for example. Diana Law describes this experience in her autobiography (Law and Paterson, 1980). At her bedside a doctor told her relatives that she would be a cabbage. Diana Law understood what was said, but could not utter a sound in protest.[1]

We also encountered some more positive feelings about aphasic living: thankfulness at being alive; gratitude towards people who help make life bearable; appreciation of valued people and things; and a determination to improve coupled with realism and the ability to take each day as it comes. Alan expresses some of these feelings: 'I would like to be a hundred per cent. I like to think about every day, not weeks or months, but every day.'

APHASIC PEOPLE'S SELF-PERCEPTIONS

Self-image is shaped by the interaction of personality factors with aspects of life that a person considers important, such as employment, family and leisure activities. A significant change in any one aspect of life is likely to lead to some modification of that self-image. Becoming disabled may affect every aspect of life, so that Paul, explaining how he felt during the months he spent in hospital after his stroke, said 'I don't think it's me.'

Having to learn to live with a 'new self' is likely to be a painful process. Bill's experience illustrates this well.

Bill lived an extremely active life before having a stroke in his early forties. He was a policeman and was married with teenage children. he had his own engineering workshop at home and a range of interests. He was keen on his work and his leisure pursuits, and a perfectionist by nature. Bill's stroke left him with severe expressive aphasia. This seriously affected his ability to read and his computational skills. Writing was affected both by the aphasia, and by having to use his left (non-preferred) hand. He could walk unaided but had little use of his right hand. His understanding and awareness were good and his memory intact. He lost his job. He was no longer able to relate to his teenage children. He took up woodwork at a social services day centre, but the results did not measure up to his high standards, so he became dissatisfied and left. At this point his self-image was a negative one; he disliked himself. He began to rebuild his self-esteem and learn to like himself again through carefully devised project work geared to his interests at a day centre for brain-injured people.

Disabled people may feel self-conscious about their appearance and about their attempts to communicate, even where relatively 'normal' communication is possible. Walter, for example, chose to attend a stroke club outside his home town, even though a similar club had been started there. He was also reluctant to shop near his home, because he did not want people who knew him before his stroke to see him disabled.

Many aphasic people, given time, do develop positive images of themselves.

Seventeen years after suffering a series of strokes at the age of 23, Mary was very capable of making herself understood, despite her aphasia. She still had some physical impairment. She led a full and active life, attending a self-help group for aphasic people 1 day a week, and pursuing various hobbies including swimming, music and pottery. She appeared self-confident, relaxed and happy.

INCOME

The impact on a person's income of becoming aphasic will in most cases depend primarily on that person's position *vis-à-vis* the employment market. The person who is retired before becoming disabled will already have established any entitlement to occupational and/or state pensions. There may still be loss of income, however, since some pensioners work at part-time 'retirement' jobs, which they are unlikely to retain if they become ill. Even if the income involved is small it might be a significant supplement to their pension. Someone of working age but not in employment prior to their disablement may depend on state benefits (e.g. if unemployed) or on the income of a partner. The question for all these people is whether they qualify for additional income from the state on account of their disability. Such income may go some way towards meeting the additional costs of disabled living.

People in employment (either employees or self-employed) will in general have higher incomes than the groups above and, moreover, incomes directly dependent on their continued ability to work. Such people, unless they recover sufficiently to return to their previous work, are likely to suffer both a significant fall in income and a change in its source. Some people who were in employment immediately before becoming disabled will qualify for income under a private or occupational sick pay or pension scheme in addition to state benefits. Their resulting income may or may not be sufficient to maintain an acceptable standard of living.

Any sudden and unexpected reduction in income is likely to have a major impact on lifestyle. Two examples illustrate the effects on families with an aphasic member whose previous income levels had been very different. Paul and his family were having to sell their holiday home at the seaside, whilst Annie and her husband could no longer afford their mortgage and had had to move to a mobile home. In her investigation of role changes following the onset of aphasia, Parr (1995) found that 'the loss of work had an impact on a range of other activities, such as travel and socializing, due to the restrictions of a limited income' and that 'financial and material restrictions are a source of concern for the majority of this sample' (p. 232).

EMPLOYMENT

Of Parr's sample, 16 interviewees were in employment prior to becoming aphasic, and 14 of them had lost their jobs. Likewise, many of the aphasic people interviewed for this book had had to give up work because of their impairment, and our overwhelming impression was that they experienced considerable regret and loss. Jack's experience is described by his wife.

He was making decisions [in his job] which affected a lot of people and a lot of money ... His life revolved around his job; his job was his life. [After his stroke] Jack's firm kept his job open for 6 months, after which Jack was examined by their doctor, and was told that he would be retired early. That to him was more traumatic, to have his job taken away, than to be told that he'd had a very severe stroke and was partially paralysed.

The impression that relatively few aphasic people in Britain return to work needs to be understood in the context of the continued high general rate of unemployment in Britain, and the fact that disabled people are more likely to be unemployed than others (Barnes, 1991; Floyd, 1991). Whether demographic or other changes will significantly affect the situation for aphasic people in the future is difficult to predict. The negative effects of unemployment, for example on health and self-esteem, are well documented (e.g. Smith, 1987) and there is no reason to believe that aphasic people escape these effects. Geoff reacted to being unemployed by sleeping all day and getting up to watch videos during the night.

There seems to have been little systematic study in Britain of the implications of aphasia for employment chances. One exception is a survey carried out by four aphasic members of a speech therapy group in Edinburgh (Dodd et al., 1992). They developed a questionnaire to tap speech and language therapists' knowledge of aphasic clients' and former clients' employment. Ten of the 22 respondents knew of aphasic people who had returned to work. They mentioned 27 individuals, 'a very small number if the therapists were thinking back to every aphasic they had treated' and 'also a small number if you consider how many people have a stroke and become aphasic in Scotland'. The findings of research on return to work after head injury are also relevant. One study of severely head-injured patients found that those who had difficulty in carrying on a conversation, or in understanding a conversation where more than one other person was involved, were significantly less likely than other patients to have returned to work (Brooks et al., 1987).

Whilst the extent and specific nature of disability are undoubtedly important in relation to employment, they are by no means the only factors. Neither can the nature and severity of the disability be considered in isolation. We now consider some other factors.

Age

Impressionistic evidence from speech and language therapists suggests that younger aphasic people are more likely to return to work than are older people. The reasons for this are probably complex, but no doubt reflect to some extent the better and more rapid recovery usually expected of younger people. It is certainly the case that priority is given, both within the rehabilitation system and by individual speech and language therapists, to any younger patients who are seen as having the potential for returning to work.

Previous job and occupational class

The findings of Brooks et al. (1987) suggested that head-injured patients' chances of returning to work varied according to occupational class. Unskilled workers were less likely than skilled or managerial workers to return. Brooks does not discuss the type of employment which returners entered, so it is not possible to judge whether this was because some disabled workers moved to lower-level employment, whether it reflected employers' attitudes, or whether it was due to some combination of these and/or other factors. There has been no comparable study for stroke in Britain, but a French survey of 63 people of working age who were aphasic after having had a stroke concluded that 'it is extremely rare that patients return to a job that is equal to the one they previously held; no such cases were recorded in this study' (Rolland and Belin, 1993, p. 227). Nearly all the returners reported to Dodd et al. (1992), however, had gone back to 'the same post or a similar post to their previous work ... Only two returned to employment in a different job' (p. 8).

The relationship between the specific nature of a person's impairment and the requirements of a particular job will be important. Professionals may be particularly disadvantaged by communication difficulties. Office work may be feasible, but interferences such as background noise and constant interruptions are likely to tire and stress the aphasic worker, whilst tasks like filing might pose difficulties. The right hemiplegia that often accompanies aphasia will probably rule out tasks requiring physical strength or manual dexterity.

Psychosocial factors

Determination on the part of the aphasic person to return to work is undoubtedly a major factor. The aphasic people in Rolland and Belin's study (1993) who found jobs 'did so thanks to their own efforts' (p. 227). These researchers' findings suggest strongly that a family's attitudes can be at least as influential, stating that:

> when patients are overprotected and considered as highly diminished (even when their symptoms are moderate), no efforts are made to help them. The family neither helped nor encouraged the person to return to work. In these cases, it is very rare for patients to reintegrate into a profession, even though they may be motivated to do so. In the inverse scenario, where families are optimistic and enthusiastic, they can

contribute greatly to the person's ability to muster and sustain the motivation essential for a return to work.

(p. 227)

The enormous range of circumstances and the interplay of different factors are illustrated by the following examples reported to us by therapists.

Len, a van driver, suffered a stroke at the age of 38. He made a good physical recovery, and returned to work. It soon became apparent that he could no longer manage his job, as he was now unable to plan a route or follow directions.

Max was a fairground stall holder who was 45 when he had a stroke. His comprehension following the stroke was good, but he was left with very little speech, just single words. Despite this, he was able to return to his stall.

Len lost his job due to his 'invisible' language disability. The factors enabling Max's successful return to work included the fact that he was self-employed, his cheerful, outgoing personality, the nature of the job, for which good understanding was essential but little speech required, the support of his wife and the division of tasks between the couple before Max's stroke (she already did all the paperwork).

Information about return to work is available from four large-scale surveys of aphasic patients carried out in Japan in 1978, 1982, 1985 and 1988 (Sasanuma, 1993). The percentage of treated patients returning to paid employment varied from 12.4 to 16.2%. Sasanuma reviews these surveys and other studies in Japan, and concludes that being relatively young, having mild aphasia and starting language therapy shortly after the onset of aphasia are correlates of return to work. Considerable caution is called for, however, in cross-national interpretation of such findings.

MOBILITY

The aphasic people interviewed for this book were by definition among the more mobile, since contact was through therapy groups and clubs. They nevertheless had mobility problems. These were due partly to the inaccessibility of much transport for people with the physical impairments that so frequently follow a stroke. Communication difficulties also played a part. Reduced mobility outside the home might, however, be less directly attributable to either motor or communication impairments. This is well illustrated by J. C., one of Parr's (1995) subjects. J. C. travelled much less than before because she had left work and had therefore lost her company car. She and her husband could not afford a new car and public transport was problematic because J.C. now had a phobia about heights.

Mobility presented fewest problems for those who were fit and able to drive. As Lebrun *et al.* (1978) suggest: 'For many [aphasic people] the car is, or at least could be, a means to feel less dependent, less diminished, and to recover an acceptable social or vocational position' (p. 56). Some people had had to give up driving and therefore relied on other people, such as spouses, friends or volunteers, to drive them, or on hospital transport. Others had come to depend on public transport. Communication difficulties such as comprehension problems might affect someone's fitness to drive. Lebrun *et al.* show that there is no simple relationship between the severity of a person's aphasia and her or his ability to comprehend traffic signs, and argue for 'an appropriate test which resorts as little as possible to language'.

Aphasia may also affect someone's ability to use public transport. For example, Alf's sister travelled with him when he went for speech and language therapy, as he couldn't find his way alone. People who had progressed to using public transport found it a cause of anxiety at first, but also an important step towards regaining independence.

People who have had a stroke often suffer from fatigue. Using public transport is more tiring than going somewhere by car, and often takes much longer. This could affect ability to work, as someone might be too exhausted to work after the journey. The same could well be true in relation to therapy and to social activities. One study of 42 aphasic stroke patients living at home identified mobility as the main factor influencing the activities these people could undertake (Smith, 1985).

EVERYDAY AND LEISURE ACTIVITIES

Of the communication-impaired stroke patients in Anderson's study (1992), a large minority (38%) 'increase[d] their social activities following stroke' (p. 169), whilst the comparable figure for stroke patients without such impairment was 15%. Anderson suggests that the main reasons for this disparity were regular attendance at social or stroke clubs by a third of communication-impaired patients, and an increase in the frequency of visits at home among this group. Likewise, Smith's study (1985) found that, while aphasia did not result in a decrease in the overall number of social contacts, the type of contact did change. Only three activities of the 12 she investigated were still performed by the majority of her subjects. Two of these – talking to doctors and to rehabilitation staff – were presumably activities directly related to the stroke. In general, contact with workmates had been replaced by contact with helpers of various kinds.

Such statistics tell us nothing about the effects of social activity on people's quality of life. We must also note that, for the majority of Anderson's communication-impaired sample (1992), social activity showed no increase. Almost a third felt that 'doing things socially, with other people, was a great problem' (compared with only 7% of other stroke patients), and over half (53%) said they had 'lost interest in things' (compared with just over a quarter of those without speech problems) (p. 169). Kinsella and Duffy (1978) found that:

> There was an almost universal picture of boredom among the patients and this was even more acute for those with aphasia. The aphasic patients not only had less to occupy themselves with, such as reading, watching television, talking with people, but had also had to relinquish more household tasks such as shopping and household business affairs.
>
> *(p. 37)*

One aphasic person, Charles, wrote: 'I can talk more easily now but I can't say what I want to and I have had to give up the things that I really enjoyed.'

Many of the people with aphasia we spoke to mentioned friends and the support they gave. Julia saw the same friends as before, and had recently become engaged. Several others commented that there were some former friends they no longer saw and that becoming disabled had shown them who their real friends were. Forty per cent of the communication-impaired stroke patients in Anderson's research (1992) felt that other people treated them differently since their stroke. The fact that the comparable figure for stroke patients with no speech problems was much lower (13%) suggests that this was due to communication impairment rather than stroke *per se*.

Nearly all the 20 families interviewed by Malone (1969) in a much earlier study said that 'their own social lives had been changed in many ways', and that 'their friends gradually stopped coming to visit' (p. 148). In many cases it was the families who had discouraged friends and avoided outings, because of their shame and embarrassment at their aphasic relative's conduct. Kinsella and Duffy (1978) found that: 'Mobility difficulties and an inherent dislike of leaving the patient alone ... meant that unless friends came to visit, there was little opportunity for social contact ... [giving] the feeling of being "a prisoner in their home"' (pp. 36–7), and that friends often stopped trying to hold conversations with the aphasic person because they found it so difficult. Activities are also affected by aphasic people's attitudes, their assumptions about the attitudes of others, what they can cope with and practical considerations. Aphasia is not always the main factor. For example, Jack's impairments made him reluctant to visit friends whose homes had no downstairs bathroom. The reduction in socializing shown by Parr's subject, J. C., seemed to result from loss of confidence and perceived changes in others' attitudes owing to her weight gain and change of self-image, which in turn stemmed, she felt, from her motor problems (1995).

Shopping and associated activities like going to the bank can present considerable problems. Aphasia may affect a person's ability to produce the names of items needed, ask their price, work out the bill and handle money. Shopping could be something of an ordeal. As George commented to us:

> I wish some people would take a bit longer time, give us time to express ourselves. Often you might be in a shop and you say something to the girl behind the counter which she doesn't understand. And rather than spend time waiting for you she goes and serves someone else.

This made it more difficult for George to find the right words. In Chapter 9 we describe attempts to ease such problems.

Many of the aphasic people we interviewed at their group were by this stage able to go shopping, either on their own or with a relative. Malcolm used a supermarket where 'nobody knows me'. Several people commented that they found shopping in supermarkets relatively easy as little speech is required. Paul's wife accompanied him the first few times he went to the shops or bank, about 18 months after his stroke. It was 'difficult at first, the speaking'. Paul continues 'and I can speak, but I can't speak, so she'd do speaking for me'. At the time of interview, he could manage on his own, except that he still got confused about 'complicated things'. Of Parr's 20 subjects, nine reported increased involvement in shopping since the onset of their aphasia (1995).

FAMILIES LIVING WITH APHASIA

To understand the effects of aphasia on families we must consider the whole family, including the aphasic member. Many such effects are illustrated above. Anderson (1992) concludes that:

> the experience of stroke is different for patients and their carers as regards attitudes, expectations, health and changes in daily life. Both groups are profoundly affected by the event but in different ways at different times ... The severity of the stroke, and of the disability, ... gives little indication of how the lives of patients and carers will be affected.
>
> *(p. 220)*

He also reminds us of the importance of 'relationships before the stroke' in understanding how families manage post-stroke (p. 216). We now concentrate on three aspects of family life with aphasia: effects of the onset of disability, changes in roles within the family and the impact of continuing disablement on family relationships.

The onset of disability

Any sudden illness is a shock that leads to a period of considerable anxiety both for the patient (e.g. Borden, 1962) and for relatives (Overs and Belknap, 1967). Alf commented that his family knew nothing about strokes before he had one; our impression is that Alf's family was not unusual in this. Words used by partners to describe their feelings include 'frightened,' 'panic' and 'uncertainty' (ADA audiocassette *Living with Dysphasia*, 1993).

The individual and family may be forced to confront the possibility of death, a subject that is likely to invoke a complex tangle of emotions. A future that may have seemed to have been mapped out is suddenly far from secure. Also life becomes centred around the patient, usual routines having to be put in abeyance. Hospital visiting times or the needs of the patient at home dictate how family members spend much of their time. This signifies an extremely busy period, which people react to in various ways. Having quickly identified her husband and children as her priorities for the weeks following her husband's stroke, Jan found that she was well able to cope and describes herself as being 'terribly organized' (ADA audiocassette *Living with Dysphasia*, 1993). Friends helped out with lifts and household tasks. Others find it 'all too much' (Norma, ibid.). Relatives may feel disorientated, and perhaps unable to take in or retain information and advice (Kinsella and Duffy, 1980).

Contact with any newly disabled person is likely to be an emotional and distressing experience, as both parties recognize and attempt to come to terms with their loss. Crying is a natural response for those most closely involved. Another common reaction is anger. Elaine remembers, as a teenager, blaming her aphasic stepmother for her disability, and Norma expressed similar feelings about her husband's stroke: 'Almost, you feel … that it's his fault' (ADA audiocassette *Living with Dysphasia*, 1993). Since using language to communicate something of our anxieties, fears and other feelings can be an important strategy for coping with them, language impairment imposes particular difficulties (Brumfitt and Clarke, 1983).

An immediate task for Jan was to tell the children:

> I told them, not everything that had happened, but … that Daddy had had what looked like a stroke, and that he was quite seriously ill. I didn't want to frighten them, and I wanted them to feel that we were still in control, that it wasn't so awful. That seemed important to me. But they needed to know it was serious. They asked lots of questions. I didn't give them all the information I had, but I gave them enough for

them to feel that they were being told ... They needed ... to be re-assured that their life actually was going to continue, as children's lives do.

Role changes within the family

Being aphasic may mean an augmented role within the family as well as complete or partial loss of some roles. By far the most frequent reason given by Parr's subjects (1995) for gains in roles was that they were 'around more'. Aphasia may involve partners taking on new roles and losing existing ones. In several instances people who had previously played no part in dealing with family finances had to take full responsibility for these when their part-ners were taken ill. George's wife, for example, had not worked for many years, and had never written cheques or checked bank statements before George's stroke. Elaine's father took responsibility for paying bills, which her stepmother had done before. Driving was another activity that a num-ber of women had had to take over from their husbands. Some wives had learnt to drive and others had to get used to driving a larger car, as the hus-band's disabilities meant that he could not get into a small one. It took one man many weeks to accept that his wife would have to drive his car.

Experience regarding spouses' employment varies. Two male carers in Malone's sample (1969) reported neglect of their jobs and greatly increased responsibility for household chores. Jim (ADA audiocassette, 1993) explains how they managed:

I was able to return to work for several years after Dorothy was ill ... Dorothy's parents came one week, and then a friend would come and look after her the next week, while I was at work ... If help is avail-able, then you should accept it. No question about that.

We also encountered aphasic men whose wives were in employment. Other women were in Beth's position. She gave up a full-time job in order to look after her husband, hoping initially to find local part-time work, but had to abandon this idea. Pam's feelings of loss and frustration are very evi-dent in her comment: 'Stroke happens within a few seconds, and within those few seconds, I was reduced from being a wife and businesswoman to being a nursemaid and a nanny.' Pam's social activities were limited by her husband's long-standing dislike of being alone and his inability to cope with the conversation that 'sitters' seemed to think was expected of them.

Disablement could involve major role changes for other relatives too, as shown by the following two examples:

Mary's children were both toddlers when she had her stroke. Her disability ended her relationship with her partner and she moved in with her parents, who brought up the children. She was very conscious of the strain that 'having to start again with a young family' had put on her mother's health.

Elaine frequently stayed away from school to look after her baby brother in the months after her stepmother's stroke. She also accompanied her to push the pram and carry shopping. She describes it as a nightmare. She was acutely embarrassed at her mother's appearance, uneven gait, poor speech and inability to handle money. She thought her mother was stupid and often 'took over' from her. Elaine was afraid that people would not like her because of her mother's impairment. She thought that people would think her mother was drunk. When she first went to work, she developed an elaborate rigmarole as to why friends couldn't come to her house. It was over a year before anybody gave Elaine even a basic explanation of her mother's condition.

Effects of continuing disability on family relationships

Many of the people with aphasia we encountered received, like Mary, a tremendous amount of support and encouragement from their families. Alf's wife suggested using a tape recorder so that he could listen to his speech, and spent half-an-hour every night working with him on his spellings. His family gave him books to read and his sister took him to speech therapy sessions as his wife was at work. Family relationships can affect ability to cope with major changes. Flowers and Korczak (1981), for example, found that: 'where the family were pulling together, finances were not seen as such a problem, or they all adjusted to the situation, even where the breadwinner role had been transferred to the wife' (p. 43).

Nevertheless, disability does create additional stresses in family relationships. Relatives may interpret an aphasic person's inability to respond normally as deliberate awkwardness (Mykyta *et al.*, 1976). One carer we interviewed, whose husband's aphasia resulted in requests coming out as commands, confessed to irritation at being ordered about. Some carers find their increased responsibility difficult to cope with, while others may be unwilling to relinquish it when appropriate (Borden, 1962). Uncertainty as to how to react may lead to excessive attention to the aphasic person or a pretence that there has been no change (Malone, 1969).

Sparkes concludes from a literature review that 'a marital relationship will be permanently altered when one spouse experiences language loss resulting from a stroke' (1993, p. 10). Malone, Ptacek and Malone (1970) used an attitude questionnaire with a sample of 30 spouses and found evidence in all cases of both 'overprotection' and 'rejection'. Kinsella and Duffy (1980) and Mykyta *et al.* (1976) also found 'overprotection' of stroke patients to be common, partly for fear of stress bringing on another stroke, or of a further stroke or a fall occurring if the disabled spouse was left alone. Kinsella and Duffy (1980) found only relatively slight evidence of rejection. Their comparison of stroke couples with and without aphasia showed that it had a significant effect on marital relationships, with aphasic people's marriages being 'characterised by problems of interpersonal communication, diminished sexual satisfaction and loss of partnership' (Kinsella and Duffy, 1979, p. 129). More recently, Anderson (1992) concluded that the main impact of speech problems lies in their negative effects on the quality of family and social relationships. He found that, at 18 months post-stroke, speech-impaired stroke patients were less likely than others to report having very happy close family relationships and more likely to say that 'there was nobody they felt close to'. More of their supporters reported that 'their relationship had changed since the stroke' and that 'positive elements of their relationship with the patient had diminished'. Female supporters of male patients 'were particularly likely to describe their relationship as not very happy' (p. 168–70).

Mulhall's detailed 'mapping' of spouses' interactions (1978, p. 132) provides, to some extent, a counterbalance to this depressing picture. His research demonstrates the 'intrinsic complexity of social interaction' and, incidentally, the danger of oversimplifying reactions into a small number of categories. He found frequent evidence that 'patients were able to offer comfort and support to relatives who had difficulty coping' and of spouses' 'attempts to help and encourage the patient', though these attempts often increased the aphasic person's frustration.

The experience as carers of contributors to the ADA audiocassette *Living with Dysphasia* (1993) provides further evidence that marriages can do more than merely survive aphasia. Factors identified include the quality of the relationship before the stroke and a conscious determination to maintain a sense of equality in the partnership. Carers describe sharing both tears and laughter. The ability to work round whatever problems arise also seems important. Strategies adopted to circumvent the language impairment include the use of photographs, pictures, maps, a 'wipe-clean' drawing board, books and games, asking questions which require a yes/no response and buying a phone with a memory. For a relationship to work, carers must recognize their needs as well as their partner's. Enlisting help can expand the aphasic person's horizons. Jonty tried drawing, Alexander technique exercises and sailing. As his wife Jan suggested: 'Rather than basing the relationship just on words, we tried to base it on activities.' At the same time, such activities give carers their own much-needed time and space.

Jim outlines some very positive changes he and Dorothy experienced as a result of her stroke:

It's changed us in so much as we're probably kinder to each other, and more tolerant, and much more caring, not only towards each other but towards other people ... I think you've got to be patient, and understanding, and also determined that the life you live is pretty well the same, as near as possible, to that you've left behind prior to the illness. And if you do this, then I rather think you will achieve far more than you ever think you will.

Relationships with children are also affected by aphasia. Prolonged absence from home (e.g. in hospital or for rehabilitation) may make it difficult for a parent or grandparent to sustain close contact with small children. Malone's sample (1969) included a small number of families with dependent children. One father commented that 'for practical purposes [his daughter] hasn't had a mother since she was 11 years old'. The daughter's perception was that she had lost her father too: 'His time was so taken up with Mother that he didn't have much left for me' (p. 150). Kinsella and Duffy (1978) reported that the frustration and anxiety associated with aphasia made couples irritable with their children. Elaine's experience in the following case study was very different.

> Elaine's dad was, in her words, a 'brilliant' father, always fair and reasonable. After her stepmother's stroke he did the washing and housework. He was very calm. Theirs was a very close, religious family, who just accepted her stepmother's disability. Elaine's stepmother recovered her speech completely, though it became temporarily impaired many years later, on her husband's death. Her physical disabilities also improved considerably. Elaine describes her stepmother as a *very* determined woman, and holds great affection for her.

We know of two women who have had a child after becoming aphasic. One had stopped attending a mother and toddler group as she thought the other mothers unfriendly, though with much help and support from her husband she was coping with the demands of a young child. Her strongest incentive in working to regain her speech and language skills was to help her son and avoid his overtaking her.

Jan describes the philosophy her family have adopted:

I think that it would be wrong to deny the sadness, and it would be wrong to deny the frustration. But ... what we've tried to do as a family, and it's worked for us, is to say: okay, Jonty had a stroke. We have a choice here. We can either spend our days looking back on all the things we can't do any more, or we can say, okay, this has happened, and it's a rotten thing to have happened, but our family is important: what *can* we do together?

Relationships are not static, but are likely to change over time as circumstances alter, or expectations are modified. For example, we heard of one aphasic man whose wife's rejection of him left him wandering the streets. His wife later became disabled and he found a new role at home helping her. Borden's suggestion (1962) that family members 'need time to adapt' perhaps implies a prediction of difficulties at first but improvement over time. Some findings (e.g. Oranen *et al.*, 1987) suggest that positive, optimistic attitudes and (self-reported) 'good family adjustment' to aphasia are early reactions to the disability that are not sustained among families with some years' experience of aphasia. Slack and Mulville's account (1988) shows swings from near despair to contentment, depending partly on the acceptability of the care arrangements for all involved. Similarly, the carers *Living with Dysphasia* (ADA audiocassette, 1993) record fluctuations in their relationships, in one instance a 'low' being brought on by the cessation of therapy sessions. These experiences raise issues of service provision and of how to achieve fulfilled lives – themes that we take up in later chapters.

ADAPTING TO LIFE WITH APHASIA

Our discussion in this chapter illustrates the complexity of reactions to disabled living and the variability of the experience of living with aphasia. Anderson's findings (1992) (for a wider sample of stroke patients) suggest some patterns according to class, gender and household composition, but it has not been possible to investigate these dimensions systematically in relation to aphasia. Nor have we attempted to consider whether the experience of living with aphasia has changed over the years. It is mainly the recent studies that go beyond describing or analysing 'problems' associated with aphasia to provide a more rounded picture. This might, however, be accounted for by changes in researchers' attitudes towards disability, especially because of the dissemination among them of social model ideas.

Parr's study (1994) provides a useful summary of some of the other dimensions involved. She asked 20 aphasic people and 14 partners to rate their life satisfaction first before the stroke and then currently. Whilst a small majority 'felt that life satisfaction had deteriorated', a number felt it had remained the same and two couples agreed that their life satisfaction had improved. The reasons interviewees gave for these judgements varied widely, and are quoted in full:

Reasons for deterioration in life satisfaction levels:
1. *Physical factors:* tiredness, volatility and irritability, life dominated by physiotherapy exercises.

2. *Material factors:* loss of work, loss of car, loss of money, drop in standards.
3. *Social factors:* restriction of social life, loss of contacts, boredom.
4. *Emotional factors:* loss of confidence, fear of another stroke.

Reasons for improvement in life satisfaction levels:

1. *Freedom from previous restrictions:* was 'workaholic' before; more time; more relaxed; 'life is slower and more laid back'; not worrying like before; free from work; drinking reduced.
2. *Family and social life:* family seems closer; partner more satisfied, partnership closer, relationship improved; people more friendly; helping people; relationship with son much improved.
3. *Enhanced sense of the value of life.*

(p. 462)

In the same study Parr also investigated how the 20 aphasic people attempted to adapt to living with aphasia. The most commonly observed or reported coping mode[2] was fatalism – expecting and accepting the worst aspects of the condition and its likely outcome; other ways of coping were escape (denial or avoidance) and optimism. The strategy adopted most was to seek help and support from others; activity to obtain information about the condition, or to bring about changes in it and taking control, were strategies used mainly by the younger aphasic people (under 65s). Three respondents were helped by enhanced religious belief, but ten others 'maintained their moderate level of involvement in religious worship, yet did not see it as a source of help in enabling them to cope' (p. 464). The aphasic interviewees dealt with becoming and being disabled in many different ways, each person having his or her own combination. A given coping mode or strategy could vary in meaning from person to person giving enormous variability overall.

The final words of this chapter belong to aphasic people themselves, speaking on the *Personal Insights* audiocassette (ADA, 1995). Chris emphasizes the importance of not trying to do too much, pacing herself and looking after herself. Jean stresses the importance of practising her speech. Even a couple of days without much opportunity to speak sets her back. Sue describes the strategy of using 'key words' to convey a message. Binday, ashamed of his aphasia for 3 years, shares the revelation of social model thinking: 'Recently I have begun to recognise that it's not my problem that people have difficulty with me having dysphasia. People had been regarding me as a dodo head that doesn't understand anything, and that is extremely difficult to handle.'

Endnotes
[1]Diana Law recovered to become an ambassador for aphasic people in

many countries and founder-president of ADA. This book is dedicated to her.

[2]We use the terms 'coping' and 'strategy' here according to Bury's definitions discussed at the beginning of this chapter.

| 3 | # What is aphasia? |

In Chapter 2 we have described how aphasia may affect the lives of aphasic people and their families. This chapter aims to describe our understanding today of the nature of aphasia, contrasting it to normal adult communication, and drawing on ideas about communication breakdown that have developed over the last century. The chapter goes on to explain recent research on brain activity and function using positron emission tomography (PET) and magnetic resonance imaging (MRI) scanning methods (p. 45) and relates the findings to clinical observations of aphasic communicative behaviour. A discussion about the incidence and prevalence of aphasia then follows.

WHAT IS NORMAL HUMAN COMMUNICATION?

The development of human communication skills has been well described and documented. It is generally accepted that it was the skill of communication between humans that made us such a successful species, able to hunt and defend ourselves effectively as a group in prehistoric times because we were able to organize individuals to work together through communication. A simple model of the elements of communication that outlines the physical and sensory skills required can be seen in Figure 3.1.

Communication occurring between two people requires, at best, both ears and eyes. The speaker has the physical attributes of normal movement of the lips, tongue, cheeks, soft palate, pharynx, larynx and respiratory organs of lungs and diaphragm. The listener has accurate hearing, and the ability to see the speaker's face, hands and body also enhances communication between them.

The speaker with mature and normal anatomy and physiology of the organs required for speech can produce syllables at the rate of 189 per minute (Hammen, Yorkston and Beukelman, 1989), a startling achievement

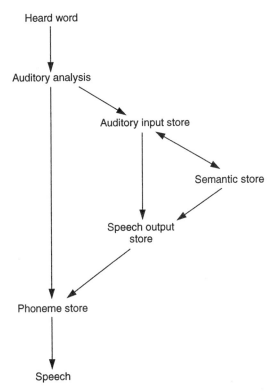

Figure 3.1 Simple model for the recognition, comprehension and repetition of the spoken word (after Ellis and Young, 1988). (Key: auditory analysis = identifying sounds; auditory input store = matching heard sounds with remembered sounds; semantic system = knowing what words mean; speech output store = matching remembered sounds with intended sounds; phoneme store = activating the sounds as words.)

of consistency of production and accurate coordination in itself. The listener must not only identify each sound produced by the speaker, but must also retain the sound sequences in order to decode the message being delivered. The sequence is important because languages have a restricted number of sounds available. English has around 50 main sounds, though of course each accent and dialect has a few of their own. As the listener breaks down the code of the sounds being transmitted into their ears, he or she is also watching the face and hands of the speaker, and paying attention to the intonation patterns coming from the speaker's larynx, which underlie the sound patterns of the articulation. The non-verbal elements of the message passed between the two are thought to carry more meaning than the speech sounds, as they relate closely to the emotions and intentions of the speaker.

The listener collects and decodes the sequence of speech sounds, deriving meaning from each word spoken and then from the sequences of the words themselves. For example, in English 'the boy the horse chases is fat' and 'the horse the boy chases is fat' contain the same words but the word sequence within the sentence is vital to convey the correct meaning. Many European languages are highly dependent on the grammatical structure of sentences for carrying meaning; however, languages such as Japanese derive as much meaning from the tones of the words as from the words themselves. So both the speaker and the listener require some sophisticated knowledge about the meaning of grammatical structure in their language before they can usefully speak or understand it.

It is at the point at which a message is transported between one person and another that one might consider that communication has taken place. And of course, in a continuing exchange of words, communication happens at a very fast rate with a very subtle exchange of meanings at the level of the words, the grammatical structures, the intonation patterns and the face and body movements of the two or more participants.

SO WHAT IS APHASIA?

'Aphasia' covers a constellation of symptoms that can cause the disruption of normal communication pathways between two or more people. In Britain two models of language breakdown are widely used to describe it.

The Boston model

One model, that developed by Goodglass and Kaplan (1983) and known as the Boston model, describes aphasia in terms of five groups of symptoms (Figure 3.2).

Broca's aphasia – awkward articulation, restricted vocabulary, simplified grammatical structure, preserved auditory comprehension
Wernicke's aphasia – impaired auditory comprehension, fluent and paraphasic[a] speech
Conduction aphasia – predominance of literal paraphasias, fluent and well articulated, preserved auditory comprehension
Anomic aphasia – word-finding difficulty, preserved grammatical structure and auditory comprehension
Global aphasia – all aspects of language severely impaired

[a]Paraphasia   – 'literal paraphasia' is a sound substitution such as 'sand' instead of 'hand';
          – 'verbal paraphasia' is a word substitution such as 'foot' instead of 'hand'

Figure 3.2 The Boston model.

A pattern of symptoms described by Goodglass and Kaplan as **Broca's aphasia** presents as a good level of understanding of speech, and an ability to produce meaningful speech, but in a non-fluent, restricted manner that removes the flow of speech. The aphasic person below (W.) is discussing how she feels her speech is that day to a student speech and language therapist (Th.). (The numbers in brackets refer to the number of seconds pause before the next utterance.)

W.   'Not so much at my best.'
Th.   'Do you mean this morning you're feeling a bit tired?'
W.   'Yes, I'm very . (3) . very . (4) . I don't know what I .. I don't know what I . (3) ooh.'
Th.   'Do you know what you want to say but you can't find the right word?'
W.   'No I can't I can't no .. not for . no not for . no.'
Th.   'And you can't get your thoughts together?'
W.   'No . no not when I .. you you good and you good(7). I can try my self .. when I'm good, when I'm very good when you come yes .. yes .. yes.'

An alternative pattern of aphasia might be characterized by limited understanding of speech, a high level of paraphasias or word substitutions and a stream of fluent speech. This pattern of symptoms would be labelled **Wernicke's aphasia**. The following aphasic person (J.) is describing what the doctor said to him about his aphasia with his wife and a student.

Wife   The doctor says he's had his stroke and he needn't come back to the clinic any more.
J.   'I just take him for to get off me .. think that was it hinny, Saturday and gauze .. city pan and er .. no.'
Wife   'He was saying to him what was his name like . you know .. couldn't say like.'

Goodglass and Kaplan described how a type of aphasia would present and also how it might recover over time. Describing aphasias as patterns of symptoms can be helpful in that patients with aphasia can be seen as part of subgroups and so some treatment patterns can evolve for managing certain symptoms. The recovery patterns expected of aphasic patients when viewed using this model are of great interest to aphasic people and their relatives. For example, Wernicke's aphasia as described above can develop into **conduction aphasia** as the client recovers skills in understanding speech. As a consequence of better understanding aphasic speakers may be able to monitor their own output and thus both anticipate and correct errors. Therefore they are able to achieve more consistently accurate speech.

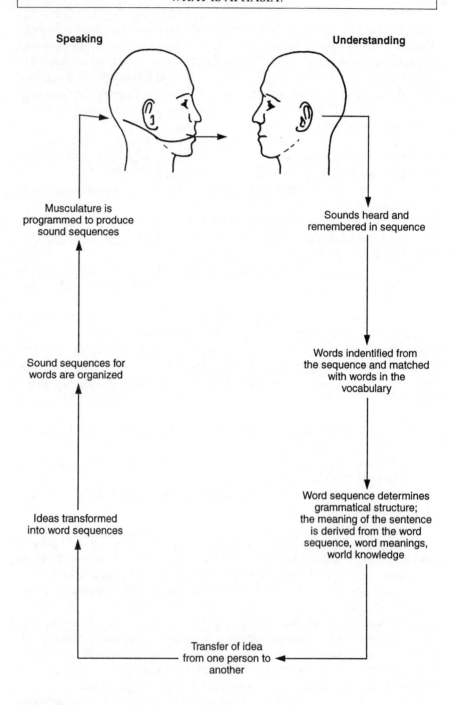

Figure 3.3 A simple model of understanding and speaking

On the other hand, patients who begin their aphasic career with patterns of communication breakdown that are characteristic of conduction aphasia may develop into an **anomic aphasia** pattern as self-correction improves.

Observing, describing and reflecting these patterns for patients and families can be extremely helpful since the aphasia takes on some predictability and some logic in its changing presentations. The Boston model describes aphasia in terms of symptoms without attempting to look in any depth at the processes involved in the communication breakdown. It does not explain why aphasic persons are unable to understand or use speech effectively, just that they do not do so.

The cognitive neuropsychological model

The cognitive neuropsychological approach, first described by Coltheart *et al.* (1987) attempts to explain the breakdown in terms of faulty processes such as, for example, difficulty in identifying one sound from another, or in identifying which sound sequence matches with which word held in the memory (Figure 3.3). It hypothesizes that there is an area of activity in the brain that interprets word meaning, and that damage to this process can cause difficulty in knowing which semantic or meaning group any word belongs to. So, for example, a semantic problem might be evident if the person were unable to identify whether a hammer was a tool or a piece of cutlery.

This approach to understanding aphasia can be helpful in determining how to develop therapy for an aphasic. However, many aphasias are complex and resist attempts to reduce them to one or two disturbed processes. Thus it is difficult to be certain that therapy is directed at the most appropriate area. For example, patients may appear to have difficulty in semantic knowledge of a word, but if they also have problems in consistently identifying sound patterns then any testing on semantic knowledge will be hindered by the preceding problem with sounds. This model for understanding aphasia has not been used widely in Britain for long enough for methods to evolve for predicting the development of the aphasia over time, and it also seems to be a very difficult model for families and patients to understand.

Although the two models can be used in a complementary fashion by clinicians, according to the needs of the moment it would be much more satisfactory to have a single model with which to describe language breakdown in aphasia, since the mystique surrounding the diagnosis and management of aphasia can be perpetuated by the lack of clarity engendered by using more than one model.

Speaking, writing, understanding, reading

The four domains of communication – speaking, writing, understanding speech and reading – are closely related in normal communication and this usually remains the case in aphasia.

The strong relationship between understanding and use of speech is illustrated by an aphasic woman named Sarah who had virtually no understanding of the spoken word at 4 to 5 years post-stroke. However, she produced a lot of 'speech', which was English sounding but had no discernible meaning in it, although she patently did mean something in her attempts to communicate in that she participated in conversation. She seemed unaware that her speech made no sense, speaking for long periods of time and then expecting a response from her listener. An explanation for this behaviour, which is frequently seen in globally impaired aphasic people, is that because she could make no sense of others' speech she was paying little attention to it. She was similarly not attending to her own speech, and therefore was unaware that it did not make sense.

This example illustrates that the understanding of speech and the use of speech are inextricably tied to each other, since understanding both of others' and one's own speech underpins any use of it. In aphasia, the general rule is that the ability to understand speech equals or exceeds the ability to use it meaningfully, at whatever level of complexity.

Similarly, understanding speech and understanding the written word are often closely linked. Whilst an aphasic person may be able to understand the written word more reliably than the spoken word at times, or vice versa, it is more common that the spoken word carries a greater meaning than the written word.

Most predictable is the relationship between speaking and writing, whereby the ability to communicate verbally is usually better preserved than the ability to communicate in writing, perhaps because prosody and gesture carry so much of the meaning in the former.

Finally, a characteristic of aphasia is its variability, even within one individual whose condition has stabilized, in that bursts of speech or periods of clarity in understanding can be followed by silence and struggle.

COMMUNICATION AND APHASIA

Earlier in this chapter a simple model of normal communication was described, referring particularly to the simultaneous nature of communication, with both partners taking equal responsibility for ensuring that ideas are passed effectively between them. In aphasia, the responsibility for effective communication can no longer always be borne equally by both partners. The non-aphasic partner is required to change his or her communication quite extensively to ensure that effective understanding occurs and coherent expression of ideas is accomplished.

Many non-aphasic partners are able to adapt their communication skills naturally and sensitively as a response to the aphasic person's communicative state, but for others it can be helpful to understand more about the processes of normal communication, and how they are transformed in aphasia, as a basis for consciously learning the adaptive skills needed to help communication work well.

CAUSES OF APHASIA AND ITS INVESTIGATION

As stated in Chapter 1, this book is largely about aphasia after stroke or cerebrovascular accident. There are four major causes of stroke:

- A thrombus is a blood clot that forms in an artery in the brain thus blocking the flow of blood. This type of stroke can occur when blood vessels are narrowed by a build-up of fatty deposits on the artery wall.
- Bleeding or haemorrhage of blood may occur from a brain artery into brain tissue; this may be caused by diseases of the circulatory system or trauma.
- There may be blockage of a brain artery by a small blood clot carried from somewhere else in the circulatory system. The tissue for which the blood is destined is starved of oxygen and there is a build-up of pressure behind the blockage. Sometimes the blockage or embolus will clear itself, in which case the effects of the blockage can be transient.
- Pressure on any part of the brain tissue or blood supply can obstruct an artery, and can be due to a tumour or swelling related to trauma.

Investigation of the site of damage

Early identification of the cause of the stroke is important since measures can be taken to reduce the area of damage, such as surgery in the case of some haemorrhages or drug therapy to restrict further bleeding in the case of others.

Various diagnostic techniques are currently used:

- **Computed tomography** (CT) scanning (available since 1972) offers an X-ray of skull and brain tissue by registering the intensity of an X-ray beam at a number of points along the path of a moving X-ray source and stationary detectors. A computer reconstructs an image of brain tissue, reflecting the presence of any damage by differences in colour.

- **PET** scanning was developed in parallel to CT scanning and uses many of the same principles to create a brain image. In this technique, positron-emitting radioisotopes form the internal energy source and are injected into the patient. Brain tissue is examined by detecting high energy gamma rays produced by the brain. Cerebral blood flow, glucose metabolism and oxygen utilization by the brain tissue can be detected. PET scanning requires a smaller dose of radiation than does CT.
- **MRI** is a very recent innovation in imaging techniques, but very expensive. The images are produced by disturbing the magnetic activity of electrons within brain cells, giving particularly clear images because brain cells, as opposed to other types of cells, have a relatively high water content.
- **Angiography** is an invasive investigative procedure requiring the injection of a contrast medium into the patient, and the passing of X-rays through the tissue. It permits inspection of the circulation of blood within the brain, facilitating the diagnosis of any malformation of the arteries and veins. It is most often used in the investigation of stroke in the younger patient and in those with minor clinical symptoms or small areas of brain damage.

Localization of the stroke and the effects on language

The Boston model of aphasia was described earlier in this chapter. The categorization of symptom clusters of aphasia into Broca's, Wernicke's, conduction, anomic and global patterns by Goodglass and Kaplan (1983) was based on ideas presented in the 1800s by the physicians Broca and Wernicke. These investigators were among the first to describe areas of damaged brain tissue as being related to specific patterns of language breakdown, their findings developing from post-mortem examinations of aphasic people with whom the physicians were familiar and whose aphasia had been relatively closely described.

The development of sophisticated examination techniques that can be applied to individuals who are not only alive but also awake and active has taken our understanding of the areas of the brain involved in communication forward at a great pace. A recent study by Peterson *et al.* (1988) used PET scanning to measure activity of the brain during single-word processing. They showed that the visual and auditory input of words occurred via multiple routes into the brain. Output that involved the processing of word meaning appeared to relate to the frontal and temporal lobes (see Figure 3.4). Speech such as repetition that required no processing of meaning failed to activate these areas.

A summary of the knowledge gathered to date on the localization of language using CT and PET scanning was undertaken by Metter (1991). He described the popular model of aphasia as being based on left hemisphere dominance for language, and that there was an awareness that left-cortex–right-cortex connections played an important role in language functioning. It was formerly supposed that sound was received and processed in the temporal lobe, reprocessed in the temperoparietal areas, and transferred to the frontal cortex for a response. However, more recent evidence has suggested that damage occurring to the deep brain tissue has caused aphasia-like syndromes and it has become evident that subcortical connections (i.e. deep connections between the hemispheres and the cortex) are also important. Metter has suggested that there are some new dimensions in brain function to be considered when describing the seat of aphasia, in that no matter where the superficial structural damage is located it may lead to chemical changes affecting function of the temperoparietal tissue. In addition, people who have suffered damage to other parts of the brain, including subcortical and prefrontal areas, also demonstrate aphasia-like features in their speech. Metter suggested that the traditional view of aphasia as being the result of damage in the temporal lobe of the left cortex was too simplistic to account for the variety observed in aphasia symptoms. First, areas of brain tissue not located near to the apparent surface damage such as in the frontal lobe and in the brainstem could be

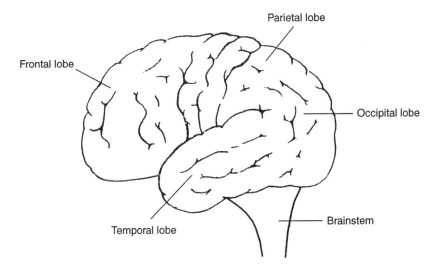

Figure 3.4 The left cortex of the brain showing the lobes of the brain and the brainstem.

demonstrated to be underfunctioning. In addition, following stroke all regions of the brain showed a depression of glucose metabolism in the acute phase of the stroke, and global glucose metabolic rates changed by 20–40% between 1 and 7 months' post-stroke in all regions of the brain.

Metters' conclusions fit with the experience of aphasia as being a widely variable and varying phenomenon. In addition, they confirm the validity of a cognitive neuropsychological approach to the understanding of the nature of aphasia, and should therefore increase our confidence in the use of this approach in its diagnosis and management.

IMPAIRMENTS FREQUENTLY CO-PRESENTING WITH APHASIA

Hemiplegia

An impairment of movement of one side of the body is termed **hemiplegia** or **hemiparesis**. A right-sided hemiplegia frequently coexists with aphasia since the brain tissue controlling the right side of the body lies adjacent to that which is most involved in language processing. However, hemiplegia and aphasia can also occur independently of each other. Where the aphasic person has been right handed, the hemiplegia can render the ability to hold and use a pencil impossible since a very finely coordinated sense of touch and control of tone in the fingers, hand and arm are required to write legibly. People with hemiplegia are often required to print large letters in their first attempts to resume legible writing, which can be slow and irksome especially where fine handwriting had been an important skill for that person. The writing impairment arising from aphasia can compound the aphasic person's difficulty in that the person initially perceives the writing impairment to be the result of the hemiplegia – in effect understood as the equivalent of having broken one's arm. The subsequent realization that movement and control of the hand and arm are returning but that the writing impairment remains can be a disturbing experience. The confusion between writing impairment due to aphasia and that due to the use of the hand and arm may be illustrated by a situation when a member of staff or family offers Scrabble letters or a typewriter to an aphasic person with a right hemiplegia, unwittingly clearly displaying the extent of the person's impairment.

Visual perceptual difficulties

A stroke that affects the performance of the occipital lobe of the brain (see Figure 3.4) may cause visual problems such as double vision, inattention to one side of the visual fields, or difficulty in interpreting visual information such as the position of one's hand in relation to the rest of the body. Some patients find that the visual disturbance interferes so much with their ability to move around that they prefer to close their eyes, relying on hearing and touch to carry out tasks.

Visual perceptual problems may not become apparent while a patient is still confined to a bed or a chair unless given help. However, they begin to interfere with the person's function as the patient relearns to wash and dress himself, and to feed himself, and they require detailed investigation, explanation to patient, family and care staff and careful management if they are not to impede the progress of the patient through recovery.

The reading impairment associated with aphasia is often misinterpreted by both patient and family as being related to a visual problem that can be resolved through a visit to the optician. Sadly, neither the visual perceptual problem nor the aphasia can be overcome so easily.

Lability

Immediately after the stroke and as a direct consequence of the insult to the brain, there can be a change in mood, which is termed **lability**. Lability is a loss of control of emotional behaviour, for instance the person may cry or laugh very easily. Sometimes crying or laughing can happen inappropriately, much to the embarrassment of the stroke sufferer, who can be aware of it but unable to stop the behaviour. Frequent crying can also be upsetting for families and care staff, who continue to respond to the person as though they were genuinely distressed. On the other hand, lability causing easy laughter can make the early days post-stroke less of a burden to all concerned. The main danger is that stroke sufferers who are prone to laughter then have difficulty having their genuine emotional needs met.

Depression

A mood change frequently observed following stroke is depression. Herrmann *et al.* (1993) identified three concepts that have been advanced in the literature to explain depression following stroke:

- aphasic stroke may result in a depressive disorder as a recognized **psychiatric** state;
- 'depressive catastrophic' reactions are a class of **emotional** reactions following brain damage;
- the depressive reaction following stroke is a natural **'grief response'**.

None of these seem to explain satisfactorily the consistent occurrence and extensive nature of depression observed in the aphasic population by clinicians.

The above authors reiterated that studies examining depression following stroke vary in their design and, most importantly, in their underlying pathological concepts so they found it difficult to draw conclusions or even establish any concurrence about the cause and nature of depression in stroke from their literature search. However, they did propose that depression may be dependent upon the course of the illness so that at each stage of recovery the aphasic person has a specific vulnerability to develop a mood disorder. They suggest that depression in the early stages of recovery may be dependent upon direct structural and biochemical consequences of the stroke. At 2–6 months post-stroke, reactive changes may occur owing to the realization of the extent of dysfunction and the slow rate of recovery. At a later stage, depression could result from a realization of the scope of physical, familial and social implications of the stroke.

A series of studies by Robinson and Starkstein (1990) confirmed that a proportion of post-stroke depressive disorders were anatomically determined, that left hemisphere damage was more frequently correlated with depressive changes and also that the presence and degree of mood disorder was related to the outcome of rehabilitation.

Coughlan and Humphrey (1982) found that a third of a group of 170 stroke patients had sought treatment for depression at 2 years post-stroke, although Währborg (1991) found that very few depressed aphasic people were ever referred for any treatment for depression. This begs the question whether aphasic people were not accessing help because it was difficult for family members to determine the extent of the problem, or because aphasic people themselves were less likely to be able to request help. Emotional withdrawal can affect communication, exacerbating aphasic symptoms by reducing the aphasic person's willingness to try to communicate by any means. Families, carers and clinicians can enable an aphasic person to locate appropriate help for depression if they are alert to the likelihood of depression occurring at any time in the recovery from aphasia.

INCIDENCE AND PREVALENCE OF APHASIA IN BRITAIN

The literature on the incidence of stroke in Britain suggests that one could expect an incidence of around 2 per 10 000 population per year and a prevalence of around 36 per 10 000 remaining disabled after stroke (Wade and Langton Hewer, 1987). Of these, 2 per 10 000 may be aphasic (Wade *et al.*, 1985), although Hopkins (1975) estimates that the incidence of aphasic survivors at 6 months post-stroke is nearer to 0.9 per 10 000.

It is still uncertain how many aphasic people there are in Britain. The College of Speech Therapists (CST) Aphasia Working Party (1989) tentatively suggested a prevalence of 150 000–200 000 aphasic people in the United Kingdom, taking all causes into account. Numbers of aphasic people in the USA have been put at 1 million (National Aphasia Association, n.d.(b) c. 1988). This would be consistent with a UK figure at the upper end of the range indicated.

It is difficult to estimate the incidence and prevalence of aphasia in Britain because:

- The incidence of stroke in the general population of any health district is uncertain unless that district keeps a stroke register, and moreover one which gathers data on cerebrovascular accident about all residents and not just those admitted to hospital.
- The diagnosis of aphasia may be unreliable unless stroke patients are assessed by a qualified speech and language therapist at the time of the collection of data for the register.
- Whilst a large proportion of people with stroke may have a communication disorder immediately following stroke, many recover rapidly and spontaneously. A proportion are left with a permanent impairment, which represents the prevalence of aphasia in the community.
- Aphasic people who obtain help from their local speech and language therapy service are thought to be just a fraction of the aphasic population in any one district, although it seems likely that those districts that are relatively well developed and organized to cater for the needs of aphasic people may well attract more referrals.

Mackenzie et al. (1993) carried out a survey of services to aphasic people across Britain during 1990–1. The survey identified a significant association between population size and number of aphasia referrals but also observed variation between similarly sized districts. For example, annual aphasia referrals for districts of 200 000–250 000 people varied from less than 50 to up to 250. Bexley Speech and Language Therapy Service, which is recognized as a centre of excellence, had a total of 101 new aphasia referrals in 1991–2 from a resident population of 221 700 (personal communication), a rate of 4.6 per 10 000. The Nottingham service, which has a stroke research unit, had 188 new referrals in 1990 from a population of 660 000 (personal communication), or 2.9 per 10 000. Newcastle upon Tyne has an annual referral rate of around 250 aphasic people from a population of around 279 000, or 9.0 per 10 000. However, Newcastle traditionally draws around a third of its referrals from surrounding districts. This information suggests that, whilst each district service may be able to keep the most accurate information about the incidence and prevalence of aphasia locally because expert assessment is available at referral, nevertheless since districts probably do not gather data on all aphasic people living in the locality the data is still fragmentary.

In this chapter we have considered the causes, nature and distribution in the population of the range of impairments labelled aphasia. This has meant focusing on the impaired individual, to the virtual exclusion of that person's 'significant others'. It is an essential component of any understanding of aphasia. It is not, however, the main concern of this book.

PART TWO

People and Policies

What is aphasia therapy? | 4

Therapy is not a prescribed response to aphasia but rather a range of aims and strategies initiated usually by a speech and language therapist to aid an aphasic person to overcome the aphasia. Therapy can be a complex, multi-faceted series of tasks and activities carried out between aphasic patient, therapist, relative and sometimes volunteer or friend. To understand these tasks and their aims as traditionally conceived by speech and language therapists, it is helpful to use the conceptual framework of impairment, disability and handicap. These terms have been extensively discussed in their application to physical impairments but discussion on how they might be applied to communication disorders such as aphasia has been limited.

Worral (1992) discussed the WHO definition of 'impairment', 'disability' and 'handicap' (Table 1.1 p. 4) in relation to aphasia. The definitions can be helpful in understanding the aims of different components of the therapy that could be offered to an aphasic person, and examples of each area of therapy will be presented below. Worral suggested that, from a speech and language therapy perspective, the 'impairment' of aphasia could be considered to be the performance of the individual on standardized aphasia tests, which describe skills and deficits in language performance. Thus scores on formal assessments such as the Psycholinguistic Assessments of Language Processing in Aphasia, or PALPA (Kay, Lesser and Coltheart, 1992) or the Boston Diagnostic Aphasia Examination (Goodglass and Kaplan, 1983) could be described as reflecting the impairment of that individual.

The same author described the 'disability' of aphasia as being the consequences of the impairment on everyday activity for that person. Examples would be the extent to which the aphasic person could continue to participate in decision making in the family, control the dog or be independent in cooking and shopping.

The 'handicap' of the aphasia was the value that the individual, the family and society attached to the disability. In Chapter 2 it was seen that aphasia leads to major lifestyle changes, and people's complex and multi-faceted responses to aphasia were explored. Some families and individuals find that they accommodate the aphasia in time, with or without help from others, and no longer experience their aphasia as distressing. Others find that the aphasia is an irritant that restricts their abilities to function as part of a family or as an individual. Yet others find that the disability continues to be an experience of profound loss, affecting their ability to take pleasure in living, and causing marital breakdown, mental health problems or severe distress.

Therapy for aphasia can be addressed at these three levels, and each is now considered in turn.

IMPAIRMENT LEVEL THERAPY

Direct intervention at the level of the impairment aims to change the performance of the aphasic person on aspects of communication that could be reflected in scores on formal tests of aphasia, which should also result in an enhanced level of communication for the aphasic person. It considers the communication disorder to be rooted in the aphasic person, and seeks to overcome it by maximizing the skills and competence of the aphasic person directly.

Impairment level therapy has been largely theory-based therapy, described as a series of tasks undertaken by the aphasic person under the supervision of a speech and language therapist. An example would be a self-administered treatment described by Marshall *et al.* (1990) in which patients were given a folder to take home that contained a matching task to complete for every day of the next fortnight. A therapist-administered task described in the same paper required the patient to match pictures against one of a choice of four written words, one of which was the correct name and the others were words related in meaning to the correct answer. Both tasks aimed to increase the aphasic person's ability to name given pictures, which was demonstrated for some, but not all, of the subjects in the study.

Another example of impairment therapy was that described by Nickels and Best (1993) whereby an aphasic patient with difficulty in naming worked with the therapist on a set of items and prompts that were the first sounds of the target words. So, each item picture began with one of four letter sounds. The patient attempted to name the picture with no help, but if stuck could refer to a card that showed the four initial letters occurring in the set of items, and use these as cues. The researchers found that this therapy produced significantly better naming for that patient on the specifically treated items, though not on other items that were not practised in this way.

Therapy can be at any level of language understanding or production, depending upon the skills of the aphasic person. The studies described above are directed at speech at the single-word level. Schwartz *et al.* (1994) describe therapy for understanding and using sentences in speech. They worked on the ability of their patients to identify the parts of sentence structures that were the action (verb), the doer of the action (agent) and the person being done to (the theme). They compared the patient's abilities to do identification and production tasks using these parts of the sentence both before and after therapy, and using both familiar and unfamiliar materials. The aphasic patients in this study varied in their response to this therapy; some improved in their speaking skills, some in their ability to understand the use of these structures within sentences. It was possible to identify that some patients retained what they had learned whilst others did not. Overall, those patients with relatively pure grammatical difficulties had the best response to the therapy, whilst those with more complex or severe aphasias benefited less.

Efficacy of impairment level therapy

This approach to managing aphasia has been the most evident in the literature on aphasia and its treatment, and thus is also the approach whose efficacy has been discussed most widely in the literature. There have been many attempts to examine efficacy of aphasia therapy in large trials where patients were randomized to 'speech therapist treated', 'volunteer treated' or 'no treatment' groups (Marshall, Tompkins and Phillips, 1982; Lincoln *et al.*, 1984; Wertz *et al.*, 1986); these have had limited success. The studies have taught us a number of things about aphasia, such as the large number of factors to consider in treatment, what patterns of recovery one might hope to observe if treatment was delayed and whether or not all people with aphasia are suitable for or will accept impairment level treatment.

As a result of the frustration ensuing from large group trials of therapy for aphasia, researchers began to search for more appropriate methods of capturing response to treatment. One of the difficulties apparent from grouping aphasic people for certain treatment strategies was that no one aphasic person appeared to experience aphasia in the same way as the next, therefore it did not seem to be appropriate to offer one treatment to all. A number of researchers proposed that aphasia was suitable for a single case study approach (Howard, 1986; Pring, 1986), which meant that each aphasia was treated individually according to professional judgement. Treatment was arranged in such a way that the patient was compared with him or herself, rather than with someone else; so, for example, the performance of the aphasic person on several prescribed tasks was carefully documented before treatment began. One task was then 'treated', while another was not. Afterwards, the tasks were reassessed to detect any change on the treated task and to confirm that no change had occurred on the 'untreated' task. Finally, the previously 'untreated' task was treated, while the previously 'treated' task was left untreated. Reassessment could show change on task performance specifically in response to attention and practice of the task. Just as significantly, it could show no change on tasks which were not addressed.

Of course, carrying out single case studies with aphasic patients proved to be a very demanding way of examining response to treatment of aphasia for both patient and therapist. There is also a continuing debate about the validity of any single case study, since the outcomes apply only to that one aphasic person and so are difficult to apply to any other aphasic patient who may present for treatment.

Another method for analysing the success of specific therapy tasks in promoting effectiveness in communication was recently described by Byng and Jones (1993). They have been developing a method of documenting the interactions in therapy between the patient and the therapist by coding 5-minute samples of therapy. The method promises to develop understanding about therapist style and how helpful it might be to particular aphasic persons, whether a specific task is helping to improve performance and which cues are most potent in promoting learning in the aphasic patient. The authors are still developing the coding system to improve its reliability between therapists and over time.

In summary, the single case study literature demonstrates clearly that impairment level treatment of some presentations of aphasia can be effective for many individuals with a wide variety of difficulties presenting as aphasia.

DISABILITY LEVEL TREATMENT

This type of therapy aims to reduce the impact of the impairment on the everyday activities of the aphasic person. It does not aim to change the aphasia, but rather to minimize the disturbance to communication between the aphasic person and the other people in his or her life.

A well-used approach to therapy at the level of disability is that of PACE, an acronym for 'Promoting Aphasics' Communicative Effectiveness', developed by Davis and Wilcox (1981). This treatment aims to improve the effectiveness of any communicative behaviour on the part of the aphasic person. The therapist sets up a situation in which the aphasic person has information to impart that is 'unknown' to the therapist. The aphasic person is able to use methods such as gesture, writing, indication of the written word or speech to pass the message. With modelling and extensive training this therapy technique can prove useful in teaching the aphasic person what is a useful approach to communication and also that means other than speech can be effective.

Holland (1991) described strategies that aphasic people might use which minimize the disability of the aphasia. These might be strategies that the individual had evolved him or herself, or they could be taught as part of a therapy programme. So, for example, the aphasic person could simplify or elaborate messages, repeat them and use a 'placeholder' such as a raised hand to signify that the speaker required time to find the word he or she was looking for. The aphasic person might learn to modify the speech of another by asking for conversation to be slowed down, for sections to be repeated or for more gesture on the part of the non-aphasic participant in the conversation. A therapeutic role for a speech and language therapist could be to help an aphasic person and their conversation partner to understand those strategies that are helpful and those that are unhelpful in any particular type of conversation or even in different venues.

Lesser and Milroy (1993) described 'conversation analysis' as a means by which to analyse dialogue breakdown using a 'bottom up' approach. That is, a clinician may record and transcribe a lengthy piece of dialogue, then examine it for the exchange of meaning between the two speakers and how the exchange was achieved. This method offers clinicians a structured, theoretically sound method of intervention for aphasic patient and conversation partner around such topics as opening and closing conversations, taking turns and repairing miscommunications.

When a clear understanding of the aphasia has been reached by the aphasic person, main communication partners and clinician, it can sometimes be of benefit for the aphasic person to join a group of other aphasic people who meet regularly to work, and sometimes relax together. The benefits of group work, which we discuss further in Chapter 9, are that aphasic people can see their own difficulties in perspective – for example that they are able to achieve something that is impossible for someone else in the group, or where they can offer to help someone else to do a task and so feel themselves a 'helper' rather than always being in receipt of help. New acquaintances and friends can be made, with a common area of concern, at a time when relationships with friends established in the time before they were aphasic may be under stress.

Group work with these sorts of outcomes blurs the distinction between working at the level of the disability or the handicap, since whilst one of the aims of such group work might be to apply strategies for communication, a benefit can be that the aphasic person moves some way to a deeper understanding of the aphasia, finding positive benefits in its presence.

HANDICAP LEVEL TREATMENT

Therapy at the level of the handicap is built upon work at the previous two levels, and can often be used to begin to rebuild skills and confidence in practical tasks. The consequent lift in confidence and skill can help to foster positive attitudes and feelings about the ability to cope with aphasia. One consequence of direct therapy might be to increase the feeling of control over the symptoms of the aphasia, such as word-finding problems or difficulty in absorbing the TV pages of the newspaper.

Counselling of aphasic people directly about their emotional response to asphasia has recently been explored by Ireland and Wotten (1993), supported by ADA. These authors were trained counsellors, one also being aphasic and the other a speech and language therapist. They worked together to offer a service exclusively devoted to aphasic people, in order to assess the value of counselling to this group. The qualitative study found that some aphasic people were unable to benefit from counselling but that many felt that it gave them time to talk and an opportunity to get to grips with their experiences and to reach a fuller understanding of the associated emotions. The results indicated a decreased sense of isolation for some, and an increased feeling of confidence. The severity of the communication disorder did not seem to impair the counselling process so much as did other factors such as earlier unresolved trauma and fatigue.

Among the recommendations of the study were that counselling and long-term psychotherapy should be routinely available to aphasic people and their families, and that counselling should be introduced to clients as an integral part of the rehabilitation and support process and not seen merely as crisis intervention.

A SOCIAL MODEL APPROACH TO TREATMENT

Kagan (1995) has recently taken Holland's approach to the development of theory-based treatment much further. Her theory starts from an analysis of two concepts: **competence** and **conversation**.

Kagan discusses several different ways in which competence is defined in our society. First, a 'competent individual' is seen as someone 'who has the ability to cope with complex situations and carry out specific tasks well'. Second, there are medicolegal aspects, in which being judged as competent gives individuals the power to make decisions about such things as their financial affairs and consent to medical treatment. Such decision-making power is an essential part of full adult status in our society. Third, 'social competence (and its perception by others) is central to the ability to participate in everyday life'. Kagan argues that:

the ability to engage in conversation is key to revealing competence. When a person has difficulty in talking and understanding what is said, it is hard to 'see' the active mind; it is difficult to envisage the capacity to make life decisions; and it is difficult to regard the person as a social being. These perceptions affect the way one is treated.

(p. 17)

Aphasia affects both the ability and the opportunity to participate in conversation (Kagan and Gailey, 1993). This means that aphasic people's retained competence is frequently masked.

Kagan (1995) describes conversation as being dual natured, being both a verbal activity and a 'vehicle through which selves, relationships and situations are socially constructed' (p. 22, quoting Schiffrin, 1988, p. 272); this signals the centrality of conversation to every aspect of life. She goes on to distinguish between **transaction** – 'the exchange of information, opinions and feelings', traditionally the focus of speech pathologists' rehabilitative efforts, and **interaction** – or 'social connection', and emphasizes that it is the interaction between the two that is of importance for communicative success. Her argument is that the role of the speech and language therapist should expand in order to address the need for balance between transaction and interaction in aphasic conversation, suggesting that direct work with communication partners, including health care professionals, is central to continuing treatment beyond its traditional limits. She suggests direct discussion of the nature of transaction and interaction with aphasic people and their communication partners, provision of structured opportunity to reveal masked competence for communication, and awareness of the need to increase the access for aphasic people to social and community life.

Kagan's description of aphasia (1995) is in accord with the social model of disability (see Chapter 1). She suggests that the definition of aphasia be extended to mean 'an acquired neurogenic language disorder that masks competence normally revealed through conversation' (p. 20), and perceives that the barrier to communication in aphasia is not only the impairment but also the limited degree to which untrained communication partners are able to 'unmask' the aphasic person's communicative competence. Trained conversation partners can enable aphasic people to participate successfully in conversation, so revealing their competence. These conversation partners thus provide a 'communication ramp' analagous to wheelchair ramps for mobility-impaired people.

This perspective on aphasia is further strengthened by the adoption of a theory-based approach, which will be familiar to speech and language therapists and may make it more legitimate to invest resources in the development of treatment strategies beyond those founded on the impairment of the aphasic individual. Just as powerfully, there may be a shift of focus towards shared responsibility and thus attention to the skills and behaviour of conversation partners as much as to the aphasic person.

The question of whether this approach is applicable to all aphasic people is addressed in Kagan and Gailey (1993). Experience at the Aphasia Centre – North York is that severely aphasic people can participate successfully in conversations provided that they are able 'to indicate yes/no accurately in some way most of the time' and 'to understand simple questions and statements in some form (spoken, written, drawn, gestured, pointing responses, or combinations of these)' (p. 210). The North York approach has been found to work far better than might have been predicted for some members who would be described as globally aphasic (see p. 40). Nevertheless, the approach is applied most easily where the main difficulties are in speaking, rather than in understanding, language, and most members of the Aphasia Centre 'have predominantly expressive disabilities' (p. 211). Kagan and Gailey state that 'Those with predominantly receptive disabilities and fluent speech require special attention ... Groups should be limited in size and should not comprise exclusively receptively impaired individuals' (p. 211). People who are already 'independent communicators' might appear to have little to gain from the Aphasia Centre, but 'their regular attendance ... attests to the fact that simply being functional is not enough' (p. 211).

ACCESS TO THERAPY

There are a wide variety of therapies available to ameliorate aphasia, and most patients in Britain should have access to all of them through their local NHS speech and language services. However, therapy will generally be offered and then maintained only if the therapist considers that the aphasic person is able to benefit from therapy. In fact, some therapies may not be offered at all if the therapist feels that concentrating on another area is likely to be more beneficial for that patient. For example, Lendrem (1994) found that speech and language therapists offered impairment level therapy to only about 30% of the aphasic patients referred in a study looking at selection for treatment in clinical practice. Those aphasic patients were chosen who were highly motivated to work in therapy and had moderate levels of aphasia. It seemed likely that the aphasic patients not offered impairment level treatment were instead offered help at the level of the disability and the handicap, but we need more studies on current practice and how this influences the services which aphasic patients receive.

At the North York Aphasia Centre, an aphasic person whose ability to benefit is in doubt attends for a trial period to enable observation 'to assess more accurately his or her ability to participate in a conversational group' (Kagan and Gailey, 1993, p. 210). The importance of motivation is acknowledged, and 'lack of motivation ... can prove to be more of a challenge than level of severity for a communication partner attempting to maintain a conversation' (p. 210). However, Kagan and Gailey emphasize the danger of deciding too early that an aphasic person is insufficiently motivated, since it has been found that 'it may take up to a year before change is consistently observed' (p. 210). This reinforces a warning given by Anderson (1992) who writes:

> Attitudes to the illness and to disability appear to have a ubiquitous influence on response to the stroke and its consequences ... The problem ... is that these attitudes ... although recognised as potentially critical for recovery ... are so often seen as personality characteristics, such as 'motivation', when they are in practice mutable and respond to a variety of conditions, possibly including counselling.
>
> *(pp. 218–19)*

We consider access to aphasia services further in Chapter 5.

OUTCOMES OF THERAPY

We have already discussed above the difficulties in reflecting progress owing to therapy using traditional research methods that require groups of aphasic people to be treated as though they all had the same problem. An alternative approach to examining the outcome of a period of treatment of the aphasia is to capture not only results using standardized tests or test–retest of performance on specific items related to therapy but also the aphasic person's opinion on whether therapy has been of benefit to his or her everyday life. There is a view that the patient's perception of the benefit of healthcare treatments is as important a measure of the success of healthcare delivery as are attempts to document changes in objective health status.

Although it is acknowledged that there are difficulties inherent in asking patients whether they felt as if an episode of health care was of benefit, there are now some tailor-made questionnaires available for health services to utilize or develop further for themselves. For example, the audit questionnaire set out by Anna van der Gaag for the College of Speech and Language Therapists (CSLT) (1993) can be completed by the aphasic person or their carer, and asks about the level of understanding of the condition, expectations of therapy, access to services, information about the condition and apparent relevance of therapy given. A follow-up questionnaire in the same manual offers the aphasic person or carer the opportunity to say whether they were satisfied with the therapy they received, and also whether they think that there was any change in the identified problem.

This type of information can be very helpful to the therapist concerned with an individual patient since it clarifies the response to the therapy already undertaken, making it clear where there may need to be repetition or confirmation that the approach so far has been helpful. On a larger scale, collecting this information gives direction to a speech and language therapy service to adjust the delivery of services so that they are perceived by the patient as being not only what they expected but also beneficial.

It has been argued elsewhere (Enderby, 1992) that it is the handicap due to the aphasia that should be the focus of any intervention, and therefore one sensitive way of estimating response to treatment would be to document the distress due to the aphasia experienced by both the aphasic person and their main carer.

These and other attempts to obtain recipients' views as part of service evaluation are to be welcomed. They have considerable potential to enhance the sensitivity and appropriateness of services. One aspect of their design can, however, be criticized from a 'social barriers' perspective. The examples described above use a questionnaire to be completed by the aphasic person or carer. It is not clear whether carers who respond are being asked to relay the aphasic person's opinions or to give their own views on services. Carers' perceptions will inevitably be shaped by their own perspective and interests. In some instances, there will be a sharp divergence between these interests and those of the aphasic person. For example, a carer may favour the aphasic person's attendance at a day hospital in order to receive therapy. This might well be important in enabling the carer to continue to cope. The aphasic person's views on the same service might be shaped partly by recognition of its importance for the carer, but will also be influenced by other factors such as the experience of day centre life and the day hospital's perceived suitability as a setting for speech and language therapy. Ideally, any help required to elicit the aphasic person's views should come from a neutral third party. If this was not practicable, any questionnaire should at least be designed so as to acknowledge the possibly different interests of carer and disabled person, and to ask explicitly for the views of each.

Capturing the degree of satisfaction or distress of the users of health services in a valid manner presents a challenge, especially where those users have a speech and language impairment. However, Lomas, Pickard and Mohide (1987) executed a piece of research designed to compare the views of speech and language therapists on the communication needs of aphasic people with the views of a number of aphasic people themselves. Lomas *et al.* were satisfied that, under certain conditions, the views of aphasic people could be elicited and documented for the purpose of evaluating services.

Voluntary organizations have a part to play in service evaluation. We would envisage an input here at local service level only where the organization was actively involved in the particular locality. A national voluntary organization would probably be in a better position to comment on services nationally than on the details of local services. National charities gain much information through the enquiries they receive and through other contacts with aphasic people and their families. One limitation is that people may be most likely to turn to such a body where services are viewed as being deficient, so charities may receive less information from consumers as to what is good about health care for aphasic people in Britain in the 1990s. There is also the danger of confusion between the views of aphasic people and those of their carers where an organization is concerned with both groups.

Evaluation demands clarity about the aims and intended beneficiaries of the services to be evaluated. Arguably, one of the benefits of the process is in increasing providers' awareness of their goals. It is also important to be clear about the aims of evaluation itself. Much of the pressure to evaluate services can be traced to the view of health care as a business. Within this conceptual framework, evaluation is a form of market research. Consumers are asked for information that may be used to modify the 'product' of health services. This information generally flows one way – from the consumer to the organization. For disabled consumers, this approach is likely to maintain the status quo, including any 'social barriers' built into the substance of services and the process of service delivery. It is important to recognize that, even within this framework, there is much genuine interest among speech and language therapists in finding out people's wants and needs in order that services may be geared as far as possible to meeting them. So patient satisfaction is seen as a valid goal in its own right, quite apart from physical outcome of therapy.

An alternative approach to evaluation sees it as a way to empower service users. Here, there is a dialogue with service users to attempt to achieve the optimum service from their perspective within predefined resource constraints. This raises the possibility of far more radical changes to services, and of dismantling social barriers that may reduce the effectiveness of services in meeting the real needs of disabled people.

5 | Models of provision for aphasia

Aphasic people will commonly experience aphasia services as one of a plethora of services, both over a period of time and at a particular point in time. We begin this chapter with a small number of case studies, to illustrate some of the possible patterns of provision and to show the complex web of services over time. Then we focus on aphasia services, considering a range of evidence about services provided by speech and language therapists, both within the NHS and outside it, education service provision and services provided by voluntary organizations.

EXPERIENCES OF SERVICES FOLLOWING STROKE AND APHASIA: ILLUSTRATIVE CASE STUDIES

Mrs A was 68 years old and had a stroke affecting the right side of her body during her sleep one night in March. When she woke in the morning she could not sit up in bed nor speak. She found this distressing but, realizing that she had had a stroke, stayed in bed. Fortunately her sister had phoned her during the morning and, on getting a confusing reply, had come round to see her and then called the general practitioner (GP), who admitted her to hospital locally. The GP was concerned that Mrs A was thoroughly assessed and treated for her hypertension, which had previously lain undetected.

Mrs A was admitted to an acute medical ward, and underwent a CT scan to ascertain the site of the stroke and a full medical assessment. She found the process of admission, assessment and installment on to the ward an unpleasant and lengthy experience, but had little choice but to accept the situation. It was particularly difficult to indicate which night clothes she required and that she felt cold and thirsty. She wanted to remind her sister to take her cat home with her and to stop the milk. The neurological examination confirmed that Mrs A had had a stroke affecting her left temporal lobe, causing her to be aphasic and to have a dense hemiplegia on the right side of her body. She was also experiencing some visual perceptual problems which made it difficult to coordinate the movements of her limbs on the other side.

After 4 days on the acute medical ward Mrs A's blood pressure began to settle down satisfactorily and she was able to stay awake for most of the day and sleep for much of the night. She was then transferred to a rehabilitation ward in the same hospital where the nursing staff began to encourage her to wash and feed herself, and to help to choose some ordinary clothes to wear instead of her nightdress. The therapists also began to work with her, asking her to try to take weight on her right side whilst sitting on the bed and then whilst moving around. She found it difficult to follow what was asked of her, not only because her limbs seemed to have a life of their own, but also because the words people spoke to her did not seem to make much sense. She needed them to repeat themselves and sometimes in the evenings it was too much effort to have a conversation at all.

Her recovery was steady and continuous. After 5 weeks she was able to stand up herself and take some steps around her bed. She was also able to wash and feed herself and manage in the lavatory, albeit very slowly and sometimes using a wheelchair when she became tired. She understood almost all that people said to her and could read the newspaper for about 10 minutes before tiring. Her speech was slow and faltering but, given the opportunity and the time, she could indicate what she wished to say. After 10 weeks in hospital she went to live at her sister's house, where her recovery continued. Her district nurse kept a close eye on her blood pressure and the condition of her skin, especially since she was sitting down so much of the time. She continued to have help from a physiotherapist who showed Mrs A and her sister how she should climb the stairs and manage in the bathroom safely. She began a programme of walking outside, which took her as far as the library and the pub though not as far as the bus stop. She had to go to see the speech therapist at the hospital weekly, enjoying the outing and the interesting people she met there but finding the taxi ride gruelling.

Six months after her stroke Mrs A was able to say that she had surprised herself in the way that she had recovered from the stroke although she had found it to be a frightening experience.

She remained living with her sister but was able to cook and do housework and they provided each other with companionship, enjoying card games.

Mr. B, who was 67 and lived with his wife, felt his right arm go numb whilst watching TV one evening. Overnight the numbness progressed to his right leg and by morning he could not speak. His wife called the GP, who confirmed that Mr B had had a stroke and that his blood pressure was very high. Rest and medication were prescribed and over the next week Mr B was cared for at home by his wife and the district nurse. Although the feeling in his arm soon returned, Mr B still had considerable difficulty in getting out of bed, moving around the house and speaking. His GP referred him for assessment at the local stroke unit; he was seen as an outpatient for assessment about 6 weeks after the onset of the stroke. Mr B attended for physiotherapy and speech therapy by ambulance twice a week for 12 weeks. Mr B had thought that he would recover his speech within about a week after the stroke but he found that 18 weeks later he was still dependent on his wife for communication in some situations, such as telling a taxi driver the destination or asking for a drink at the bar. His speech had become more fluent during this time, however. He had been able to enjoy reading despite the aphasia, but his writing remained restricted to his name and address. A year after his stroke Mr B was able to walk around the house and largely care for himself, although he did frequently feel anxious especially if his wife was out for more than an hour or so.

Mrs C was 83 and lived alone in a first floor flat. She had gone into town to do some shopping and had felt ill. Someone had taken her to the accident and emergency ward from where she was admitted to hospital for investigation. She felt dizzy and weak, and her speech seemed to be 'mumbling'. Her right arm then became numb and limp, and her face was immobile on one side. The staff on the acute medical ward diagnosed a stroke. After 3 days she felt relatively well and wished to get home to see to her dog. She went home with the services of the stroke discharge team who arranged her care in conjunction with the GP and her family. A home carer helped her to wash and dress at first and did shopping for her since her family were all working full time. Her daughters alternated cooking her evening meal for her.

The occupational therapist and physiotherapist worked with her to find ways around the problems she had in managing everything with her left hand, and to regain full movement in her

right arm and hand. The speech therapist helped her to understand why she had difficulty following a conversation or reading
the paper. The discharge team worked with her and her daughters
for 8 weeks, after which time she was able to care for herself and
her dog alone. It was another 3 weeks before she plucked up the
courage to use the bus into town again since she was anxious that
she wouldn't be able to talk clearly to the bus driver and shop
assistants.

Mr D was a 49-year-old car salesman with a teenage family who
became aphasic and lost the use of his right side whilst out for the
evening with his wife. He was admitted to hospital from the
restaurant, where he was confirmed as having had a stroke. He
had very little speech other than 'yes' and 'sorry' for around 10
days after the stroke and his right side remained numb and with
very little power. He needed the help of two nurses to stand. He
was quite distressed, particularly by his inability to speak to his
wife and sons, although he was quite resourceful in finding other
ways to communicate with them such as pointing and attempting
to write. After 5 weeks in hospital he still was not able to move
around the bed without help, and because of his age he was
deemed suitable for inpatient rehabilitation at a residential stroke
unit that had been developed in a town 15 miles from home.
  The unit offered intensive rehabilitation for an 8-week period
during which time he would also have access to counselling
services and he and his wife could participate in a support group
there. The unit would aim to get him home with support services
at the end of that time.
  Mr D found it uncomfortable at first to move from the
hospital ward to the environment of the rehabilitation unit – partly
because he was expected to do as much as he could for himself
straight away. However, the rehabilitation team quickly developed
a work programme with him that enabled him to see what his
goals for each forthcoming week would be and who would work
with him. This was a highly organized programme, which was
demanding but also supportive both for him and for his family.
Eight weeks of intensive work with weekend breaks to ease him
back into family life enabled him to return home eventually. He
used a wheelchair around the house for a while but the community physiotherapist who took over his care on discharge from
the unit took him back up the stairs after another 3 weeks at home.
His aphasia also responded to therapy. On his return from the
stroke unit he was able to converse well although he sometimes
had word-finding problems when talking to visitors. He was

unable to return to work as a car salesman since he felt his speech was unreliable under pressure although he was able to continue his hobbies of bird keeping and bridge, which he resumed with his wife on his return home.

Having used the above case studies to 'set the scene' we now change our focus. We concentrate specifically on aphasia services, and draw on evidence about their provision to enable some generalizations to be made.

NHS APHASIA SERVICES

Here we are concerned with identifying patterns of NHS provision for aphasia and variations in these patterns, and with identifying good practice. It is important to distinguish between two complementary approaches to the study of services. The first looks at services from the provider's perspective. This will answer questions about variations in types and quantities of service. For example, whilst all services in Britain provide individual therapy only some provide group therapy. The length of group sessions will vary, and some services run more than one group a week. The second approach starts from the service user's point of view, and considers the distribution of services among recipients, answering questions as to who receives what service, when, where and how.

Only since the latter half of the 1980s have there been attempts to collect systematic information about aphasia service provision. Rossiter and McInally (1989) carried out a statistical survey in eight of the 14 English health regions in 1986–7. This revealed a 'geographical "lottery of care"' (p. 6). A more comprehensive national study was conducted in 1990 (Mackenzie *et al.*, 1993). This involved a two-part postal questionnaire. Part 1, covering district characteristics, staffing and referrals, was completed by 78% of (then) District Therapists in the UK. Part 2 was concerned with practice issues and was completed by aphasia therapists who received the questionnaire via their district therapist. A total of 922 aphasia therapists were identified by district therapists and 90% of districts returned at least one completed Part 2 questionnaire (total 571).

The most recent source of information is the ADA *National Directory* (1995). It is important to note that this differs from other sources in that data has been gathered primarily to enable ADA to refer enquirers to services in their own locality, rather than for research purposes. Speech and language therapy managers were asked to indicate what services they currently offered. Information about staffing and population served was also requested. Our discussion relates to England and Wales. Information was obtained from a total of 211 self-identified aphasia services. It is the first attempt to gather nationwide information on aphasia services since the

1991 reforms of the NHS (see Chapter 6), and entries reveal something of the organizational patchwork of services now operating. Speech and language therapy services appear to be provided mostly by NHS community trusts, which contract to provide a speech and language therapy service to acute hospitals. Our impression is that only a minority of acute hospitals employ at least some of their own therapists. The information in the *Directory* is somewhat uneven in its detail, with some categories being subject to variations in interpretation. It must therefore be treated with caution. It is nevertheless a valuable source, especially as it is the first attempt to obtain details of some aspects of provision, such as private aphasia therapy. It also gives some insights into current ideas about speech and language therapists' role in aphasia treatment.

The above sources all provide mainly quantitative information for a large number of services. Jordan (1991, 1994 and unpublished research) adopted a more qualitative approach, studying services in just three districts in some detail in 1987–8 and returning to the same districts in 1993. Further research in 1993–4 by Kaiser and Jordan (unpublished) focused on people's pathways through aphasia services. Speech and language therapy managers of ten self-selected services were each asked to chart the route(s) of aphasic people through their service, identifying decision points and criteria. Overall, our knowledge from these sources is heavily biased towards the provider perspective and there is still a great deal to learn, especially from a user-based standpoint.

Increased fragmentation of services that were previously organized on a district or area basis (Chapter 6) means that we are less likely to be able to gather the sort of information collected by Mackenzie *et al.* or by ADA in the future. The influence of the professional standards document *Communicating Quality* (CSLT, 1991) on standard setting and monitoring and the intelligence requirements of quasi-markets might however mean that the information available is of better quality, if only one knew who to ask!

Staffing

Enderby and Davies (1989) recommended, for adult neurological services, a ratio of seven whole-time equivalent speech and language therapists per 100 000 population. Mackenzie *et al.* (1993) found neurological staffing levels in all districts well below this ratio, with an average of 0.94 per 100 000 population and the maximum as 3.1 (p. 46). All our sources tend to confirm the uneven distribution across the population of speech and language therapists working with aphasic adults. Mackenzie *et al.* (1993) also report 'remarkable variations in neurological staffing in similarly sized districts'. They conclude that 'contrary to the recommendation of *Communicating Quality* (CSLT, 1991, pp. 99, 104), many therapists in adult neurology neither specialise in this field nor have access to a specialist' (p. 57).

It has not proved possible to glean more recent staffing information from the ADA *Directory* (1995). One of the problems here is that it is not at all clear in many instances whether therapists' time is split between different contracts and whether hospital and community services in a given district are provided by the same body. Any effects of different permutations on continuity of care for patients are also impossible to judge. It may be that as the number of speech and language therapists in any given area is very limited, the NHS changes have affected mainly the transfer of money and have had less impact on who treats which patients than one might expect.

A minority of services employ speech and language therapy assistants in aphasia services. The 1993 study of Mackenzie *et al.* found 20% of districts with assistants working in aphasia services in 1990. The ADA *Directory* shows 32% of services as having at least one assistant. Some of these may work in other parts of adult speech and language therapy services, but even this might benefit aphasia services indirectly by freeing some therapist time. Two services mentioned employing a bilingual assistant (ADA, 1995). Only a very small number of assistants worked in any one department and many assistants were employed part-time so, overall, their input to aphasia services is likely to be very limited.

Locations of care and access to speech and language therapy

Aphasia provision has developed as a predominantly hospital-based service. A service for acute hospital inpatients and outpatients is provided in all parts of the country, whereas services in aphasic people's own homes, residential care homes and community settings such as community hospitals, day hospitals, health centres, GP surgeries and social services day centres are less universally provided (Mackenzie *et al.*, 1993; ADA, 1995). Of services with entries in the ADA *Directory,* 87% claimed to offer a domi-ciliary service and 82% a service in residential care settings. In each case, however, almost a third qualified their entry, for example, stating that the service was provided only occasionally, or that it covered only assessment, or assessment and advice. Under 60% offered any community-based service whatsoever, and many respondents cited one or two locations, though a small minority were offering services in a wider range of community settings.

It must be emphasized that the above statistics tell us more about policies on location of services than about practice on the ground. They show that a service of some kind is considered appropriate in a particular type of location, but tell us nothing about the quantity, quality, or nature of that service, let alone about access to the service for individual aphasic people, or even for groups such as those in residential care. These features will depend on professional judgements made with reference both to patients' needs and to resource availability. Such judgements are made at different levels. These include:

- Judgements by purchasers in specifying contracts; here, the term 'purchaser' is beginning to include some proprietors of private residential establishments as well as health commissioners and GP fundholders.
- Clinical judgements about individual patients' needs presumably made primarily by doctors in hospital and general practice, with support from nurses and perhaps other health workers. As suggested in Chapter 3, the findings of Mackenzie *et al.* (1993) probably connote a considerable amount of non-referral of aphasia. This was certainly the belief of their District Therapist respondents, only 16% of whom 'considered that they received all potential aphasia referrals'. Non-referral was blamed by nearly three-quarters of district therapists on low medical priority, with low staffing, speech and language therapy's low profile and infrequent referral from GPs all being cited by large minorities of district therapists. We discuss further this last issue of GP (non-)referral in Chapter 6.
- Decisions made by speech and language therapists responsible for managing services, many of whom say their staff offer therapy 'as and when required' (ADA, 1995).
- Decisions of those 'front-line' staff themselves about the management of their own time. As many as 49% of aphasia therapist respondents of Mackenzie *et al.* (1993) 'felt unable to offer treatment to all aphasic patients for whom it is appropriate' (p. 50).

In the past, the most reliable route into receiving a speech and language therapy service was from a hospital bed. The current trend to close many long-stay wards (see Chapter 6) is likely to mean a reduction in the proportion of people with language disorders reaching speech and language therapy from this source; a decline in hospital-based therapy; and the discharge of some potential clients to residential and nursing home care.

The apparent priority given to hospital-based aphasia services extends to the speed of response to referral and frequency of treatment (Mackenzie *et al.*, 1993). Inpatients tended to receive much quicker attention and more frequent therapy than outpatients, who, in turn, fared better than people needing a domiciliary service. Our impression is that, where community settings are available, they are viewed as an extension of outpatient clinics. We take up the issue of speech and language therapy in residential care later in this chapter. Kaiser and Jordan (unpublished data) found several service managers who were making an active attempt to ensure equity in treatment regardless of source of referral. One district service had been reorganized explicitly to achieve this end. Another addressed the problem of balancing the demand for inpatient services and the needs of patients who required services at home by developing a separate community service for adults with acquired neurological disorders. A parallel community physiotherapy service existed there, serving the same client group.

All ten services in our 'pathways' study offered **assessment** as soon as was possible, though for outpatients and domiciliary patients their wait could be as long as 3 months. Some commenced therapy straight away, giving the customary priority to inpatients. Three of the ten districts, however, required patients to wait a further time (up to 6 months) for treatment. They explained that they delayed therapy until patients were neurologically stable, thus aiming to use the speech and language therapist's time most effectively. This philosophy has developed from papers such as that of Wertz *et al.* (1986) on the comparative effectiveness of early and deferred treatment. It means that inpatients receive assessment and advice only, while resources for treatment are concentrated on outpatients. One service had developed a two-stage assessment process in which all referrals, whether from hospital or community, were classed as equally urgent. This prevented prioritization based on custom, practice and other professionals' expectations, rather than on need. Each new patient was interviewed with their carer by a speech and language therapist. The patient then entered an assessment group for up to about 3 months post-stroke, before starting individual treatment if appropriate. Patients considered suitable for individual treatment thus waited, but were offered the supportive environment of the group in the interim. Patients' ability to attend the group would, of course, depend on where they lived, whether they could travel, and access to transport. Patients assessed as unlikely to benefit from direct treatment were offered access to a self-help group or ongoing contact with the speech and language therapist for review and continuing counselling. This assessment model has been described in some detail because it addresses patients' and their families' needs for information and support at an early stage whilst rationing clinical resources for maximum effectiveness.

Lendrem (1994) examined practices in **selection for treatment** for aphasia. The research demonstrated that clinicians selected aphasic patients who were moderately affected in terms of severity of aphasia, and were highly motivated to commit themselves for a period of active treatment. Clinicians also appeared to consider the communicative needs of patients in their judgements of whether to offer therapy or support and advice. Selection is essential because resources are limited and therapists have to make decisions about the rationing of health care. Overt discussion and agreement within a speech and language therapy service about the outcomes of assessment and consequent decisions about selection for active treatment may be a means of maintaining equity of provision. Otherwise, access to therapy may depend to some extent on which member of staff carries out an assessment or on whether the service happens to have long waiting lists at the time. Pressurized services are less likely to offer speech and language therapy to patients whose ability to benefit from therapy is in some doubt than are services for which supply and demand are in equilibrium. Several of the services in our 'pathways' research (p. 71) held regular staff meetings to discuss referrals and to prioritize cases, seeing this as an important part of service management. It was especially valuable in services with a high proportion of relatively less experienced staff.

Selection will exclude some individuals and maybe also certain groups of aphasic people from direct treatment. One therapy manager participating in our 'pathways' study suggested that patients who suffer compounding difficulties, such as mental health problems, are thought less likely to gain any benefit from a restricted amount of input and therefore are at a disadvantage when competing for staff time. The exclusion of patients who have both neurological and mental health problems (a policy a number of services adopt according to the 1995 ADA *Directory*) is likely to inhibit any development of interest and skills to manage such cases among staff. It therefore seems likely that some aphasic people stand to move directly from the acute stage to that of coping with continuing disability, so missing out on rehabilitation at least as far as communication is concerned.

Access to some or all aphasia services may also be affected by factors such as proximity of the aphasic person's home to a treatment centre or group meeting place, and the availability of transport, which may mean the ambulance service, public transport, a voluntary transport service or a private car. In discussing the limitations they found in domiciliary services, Mackenzie *et al.* (1993) suggest that 'the publication of comparative costings for transport *of* clients versus transport *to* clients is long overdue' (emphasis in the original). Jordan (1991) found many deficiencies in accommodation, including a clinic inaccessible to elderly and physically disabled clients and considerable extraneous noise in therapy rooms. Some, but not all, of the accommodation problems identified had been overcome by the 1993 follow-up study (unpublished). The importance of these external factors is perhaps indicated by the 39% of respondents of Mackenzie *et al.* (1993) who 'cited access difficulties as a discharge criterion'.

Range of therapies and case management

The core position in aphasia services of **individual speech and language therapy** will be apparent from Chapter 4, where we discussed some of the main strands of current thinking about the nature and content of aphasia therapy. There has been no systematic collection of evidence about day-to-day usage of the therapeutic techniques discussed or as to 'who receives what' as regards intensity of treatment and different therapeutic strategies.

The ADA *Directory* (1995) shows that some services are unable to offer more than weekly speech and language therapy to any patients. This is contrary to the recommendations of the CST Aphasia Working Party (1989) and *Communicating Quality* (CSLT, 1991) that intensive therapy, defined in the latter document as at least three 1-hour sessions a week, should be made available, if required, everywhere. Four of the ten mainly urban districts studied by Kaiser and Jordan (unpublished data) offered intensive therapy. Only just over a quarter of entries to the ADA *Directory* (1995) indicated the availability of intensive courses. Our impression is that intensive therapy is most lacking in rural areas.

There appears to be little research addressing directly the efficacy of intensive therapy versus weekly or less-frequent therapy. One exception is a small study comparing the same ten patients' progress after a 3-month residential course of therapy with that during the preceding and following 3-month periods of non-intensive therapy. It found that 'these patients with a diagnosed condition of chronic Broca's aphasia made significant progress in speech ... during the period of intensive therapy but not during the two periods of non-intensive therapy' (Brindley *et al.*, 1989, p. 703). Furthermore, the progress made during the period of intensive therapy was maintained during the second 3-month period of non-intensive therapy.

There is an understanding in at least some European countries (Basso, 1993; Huber, Springer and Willmes, 1993) and the USA (Peach, 1993) that intensive aphasia therapy is indicated for some patients. The theoretical justification for intensive regimens tends not to be spelt out, which might suggest that it is 'received wisdom'. Different modes of funding undoubtedly have an impact, with insurance-based systems financing a finite programme of therapy for insured patients who are assessed as likely to benefit. As noted above (p. 73), in the United Kingdom therapy is traditionally much less frequent for patients outside hospital than for inpatients, for whom short, frequent contacts are common practice. For others, 'once a week' therapy was common in the past, but it is increasingly believed that this is inadequate.

In some areas therapy is offered on fixed-term contracts. These may or may not be renewable, depending on policy in each service. One department offers blocks of 12 sessions spread over between 4 and 12 weeks, after which the patient returns to the waiting list (ADA, 1995). Another delivers treatment in contracted bursts of 6 to 10 weeks (Kaiser and Jordan, unpublished data). Fixed-term contracts can be more than simply a rationing device. They arise also from the desire of therapists to be clear and open with patients about what they can offer, and about what the patient can expect to achieve. Clarity about the possible outcome of a period of therapy gives patients the opportunity to develop realistic expectations, and thus increases the chance that they will feel satisfied with their achievements through therapy. The process of setting up the contract can be useful in persuading therapists to be clear about aims (their own and the aphasic person's). This in turn enables more-focused therapy, which is likely to mean more-effective therapy. Having a pre-established end-date for therapy may also sharpen clinicians' awareness of aftercare needs, and increase their willingness to refer patients on to other services. If well done, patients should finish any given period of therapy with a feeling that they have achieved at least what they expected to achieve. A crucial factor for such an outcome is a frank exchange at the point of decision about the aims of an episode of care, both about the likely outcome and about the feelings of the patient and family thus engendered. Sensitively used, contracts with patients can be a means of setting expectations, which is as important for a less-experienced therapist as it is for a newly aphasic patient, and therefore of attempting to ensure that no one feels a sense of inadequacy or failure in what can be an extremely demanding and risky venture together.

Some provision of **group therapy** was registered in 75% of districts surveyed by Mackenzie *et al.* (1993) and in about 80% of entries to the ADA *Directory* (1995). The predominant pattern was of weekly group sessions for outpatients (Mackenzie *et al.*, 1993). In some instances, it was indicated that group therapy was offered as part of individual treatment plans, as discussed in Chapter 4. A group would be set up for a particular few patients for a limited period of time. Such a group would have specific therapeutic purposes and would cease to exist once these had been achieved. In some services, groups are run on a more permanent basis and must therefore be viewed as a management strategy. The implications of this for aphasic people will vary widely.

Some areas have adopted a pattern of service whereby individual therapy is discontinued fairly early and patients are transferred to a group run by a speech and language therapist (or at least with close speech and language therapy involvement) with the help of volunteers. Such groups are usually weekly, for a half or whole day. Some, if not all, aphasic people in the group will be assessed as having the potential to make progress. The continuing existence of the group may depend on the availability of a particular therapist. Such a service model may be more in the interests of economy than of individual patients; whether that is so depends on the extent of clinicians' involvement and the nature of the work done in the group.

Clinicians emphasize that individual therapy and group therapy serve different purposes. There are many examples of good practice based in a permanent group. Perhaps the best known is the aphasia day unit at Queen Mary's Hospital, Sidcup in south London. The unit serves as a location for individual as well as group therapy, offering up to four sessions a week where considered appropriate. Another model is for an intensive therapy group to run for a week or more perhaps once or twice a year. At least one service took advantage of the lull in paediatric work during the school holiday period to run such a group.

Speech and language therapists in Britain are strongly orientated towards promoting functional communication, that is, to help aphasic people communicate in their day-to-day lives. This may be one impetus for setting up groups and also for interest in **augmentative and alternative communication aids** including, for example, signing systems such as AMERIND and MAKATON. There are six specialist Communication Aid Centres in Britain. The extent to which they see aphasic people as among their main customers varies considerably, with one specializing in 'high tech' aids of little value to aphasic people, whilst another is also concerned with simpler aids such as signing systems and communication charts. A project at one communication aid centre employs a speech and language therapist who recruits volunteers to help communication-impaired people use their aid in everyday life.

The use of **computers** in aphasia treatment has been a growing interest among some clinicians in recent years. Just over 40% of services count a computer centre in the additional support they can offer aphasic people, though some commented that what they could offer was limited (ADA, 1995). Some departments had their own computers, whilst others had access through another body. Communication Aid Centres were one resource. The south-west of England was particularly well served in this respect, with many departments across a wide area referring to the Frenchay Communication Aid Centre in Bristol.

Mackenzie *et al.* (1993) asked aphasia therapists about **additional forms of support** available alongside aphasia therapy and for patients not receiving therapy. Social clubs were cited by about two-thirds of therapists for both therapy and non-therapy patients. Their use for the latter was associated with relatively poor speech and language therapy staffing for neurological disorders. Other types of support surveyed – counselling, relative support groups, volunteer-administered activities, assistant-administered activities and speech/language/literacy groups run independently of the speech therapy department – 'were all apparently made use of more for treated patients' (p. 53). The vast majority of aphasia therapists used at least one of the six supports. Therapists treating patients at least three times a week tended also to have available a greater number of additional support services, increasing the gap between overall levels of aphasia services in different districts. Availability of most of these support services is discussed in more detail elsewhere in this chapter and in subsequent chapters. One type of support service, counselling, we consider here.

Forty per cent of Mackenzie *et al.*'s aphasia therapist respondents could offer a counselling service to patients being treated and just under 20% to non-treated patients. Therapists in districts with more neurological sessions for their population size were more likely to offer counselling to treated patients, though it is not clear who actually provided the counselling. The ADA *Directory* (1995) suggests that counselling is available to aphasic clients in about 45% of services and that it is provided by a wide variety of agencies. Some counselling is provided by speech and language therapists themselves. Entries reveal a measure of agreement that speech and language therapists have a role in relation to clients' psychosocial needs. Some departments said counselling was unavailable, but commented to the effect 'except for that offered by speech and language therapists as part of therapy sessions'. Others said it was available, provided by speech and language therapists as part of their ongoing clinical responsibilities. This seems to suggest some uncertainty as to what constitutes 'counselling', or it might reflect the fact that counselling qualifications are held by some speech and language therapists.

All the districts in our survey (Kaiser and Jordan, unpublished data), expressed the view that continuing care for people with aphasia was a responsibility that to some extent lay with speech and language therapy services. Just under 30% of departments in the ADA *Directory* offered a speech and language therapist-led support group, but it is not clear to what extent these were post-therapy groups. One manager in our survey felt that other bodies such as voluntary organizations and self-help groups could meet aphasic people's long-term support needs more effectively. The Stroke Association's major contribution in this respect is discussed later in this chapter, and in Chapters 7 and 9. Self-help groups are a relatively new development; just over 20% of departments indicated access to such a group, rising to a quarter if groups being planned are included. We discuss the emerging role of self-help groups in Chapter 9.

It is important to consider aphasia services from the perspective of the recipients, who are likely to be seeing a number of different health and social services professionals concurrently. Speech and language therapists may work as members of multidisciplinary teams, whether in acute hospitals or in community settings. The effectiveness of services can be improved by co-operation among professionals. To take one very specific example: an occupational therapist and speech and language therapist might be working with an aphasic patient on, respectively, the identification and naming of body parts. If both therapists encourage the patient to move and name body parts simultaneously, this will provide more opportunities to practise both tasks.

Multidisciplinary settings can, however, constrain speech and language therapists' control over who they treat, when and where. A stroke rehabilitation unit may seek out patients who can benefit from the attention of the whole range of clinical staff working there, therefore admitting someone with a range of problems following stroke in preference to an aphasic person who has no perceptual or mobility problems. The speech and language therapist may well be expected to treat any communication-impaired patients admitted to the unit, regardless of whether their needs would lead them to be assessed as suitable or a high enough priority according to the prioritization system operating within the speech and language therapy service. Individual therapists may not be in a position to discharge from their caseload any patients still in the unit. Conversely, therapists may find patients discharged from the unit before the natural conclusion of the episode of therapy is achieved, either because the length of time in the unit deemed appropriate by the purchaser has elapsed, or because patients' other needs have largely been met. To some extent these problems might be overcome by sending advice and further work home with the patient, and by liaison with community speech and language therapists. It is worth noting that a conflict of interest may arise here where the home district is covered by a different provider. Sending work home could be construed as divulging information about treatment that could benefit a competitor! The above points reveal some of the shortcomings in the NHS quasi-market system (see Chapter 6) as it affects rehabilitation services.

Mackenzie *et al.* (1993) identified a small number of districts (7%) meeting every one of a range of 15 criteria derived from *Communicating Quality* (CSLT, 1991) for a comprehensive aphasia service. They were surprised to find that:

- 'Relative to population, these districts devoted no more sessions per week to the neurological caseload than districts which did not provide such a complete service' (p. 59).
- Despite intensive therapy (at least three sessions per week for inpatients and outpatients) being one of the criteria, and therapists working only a few sessions per week in adult neurology finding it difficult to offer this degree of intensive therapy, the aphasia caseload was nevertheless distributed among many therapists in these 'exceptional' districts.

The same authors explored several hypotheses to explain these unexpected findings, including limitations of their data, differing views as to optimal intensity of aphasia therapy and the use of management strategies such as skill mix and the sharing of particular patients' care among part time aphasia therapists. Further investigation is called for in relation to strategies to maximize cost-effectiveness.

Carer support

Over 90% of the respondents of Mackenzie *et al.* (1993) offered some form of carer support. Carer groups were available in just under half of services supplying information for the ADA *Directory* (1995). These were provided by a range of agencies, including The Stroke Association and more general organizations for carers. A study some years ago of a stroke relatives' support group in Australia (Mykyta *et al.*, 1976) suggested that partners of aphasic people may have a particular need for such a group. Participating staff ranked 'problems arising from communication difficulties' as the most frequently discussed issue, and comment that 'two-thirds of the relatives who have chosen to attend have dysphasic partners' (p. 89). In Britain, some groups are offered by speech and language therapists specifically for relatives of communication-impaired stroke people. It is possible to distinguish between two models: an open-ended 'drop-in' facility and a more structured 'short course' for relatives. Each may enable the dissemination of information and an opportunity to share experiences. Rice, Paull and Müller (1987) studied the effects on carers' well-being of a 'course' type relatives' group held over 12 weeks . They concluded that: 'The results ... suggest strongly that participation in a support group can be of psychological benefit to spouses of aphasic patients' (p. 254). Furthermore, there was some evidence that 'the partners of those spouses attending ... made more significant improvement than those not attending the group' (p. 254), though it is recognized that this finding is subject to different causal interpretations. One of the present authors' experiences of running relatives groups (Lendrem and Stamp, 1985) suggested that a group run jointly with an occupational therapist or social worker was better able to support carers than one provided by a speech and language therapist alone.

Another finding of this research was that only a small percentage of carers were able to benefit from meeting with other carers. This suggests the need for a variety of methods of providing support for families. Speech and language therapists will expect to give information, advice and support to relatives on an individual basis. In Sweden, Wāhrborg and Borenstein (1989) report using family therapy techniques to positive effect. We describe voluntary sector initiatives in Chapters 7 and 9. Local 'carers panels' that have been set up by purchasers in some areas would seem to be a useful source of expertise on carers' service needs. This model has been used in other areas of health care, for example in relation to carers of people with Alzheimer's disease in Newcastle.

Aphasia services in residential care

In the main, speech and language therapy services for people in residential settings other than long-stay hospitals have been underdeveloped in Britain. As Gravell (1988) states: 'It is not usual for speech therapy services to be available within old people's homes, which has resulted in staff and residents being left to cope alone, or occasional patients being transported to the speech therapy clinic' (p. 117–18). In the first of two rural services studied by Jordan in 1993 (unpublished report), people living in residential homes were treated as requiring a domiciliary service. The other had insufficient resources to provide any service at all for people in residential care. The responsibilities of one community speech and language therapist in an urban area in the late 1980s included six long-stay hospitals, a convalescent hospital (which had a steady stream of aphasic patients) and 52 residential homes. Institutions the researcher had not managed to visit were still, in effect, without any speech and language therapy service. Nearly half (48 of 102) of her (predominantly aphasic) referrals during 1 year were from institutions *following contact initiated by her*. The community therapist's workload thus reflected where she had worked rather than the actual pattern of need.

Referral to speech and language therapy will depend on recognition that the problem is a language one that is susceptible to treatment. A project in Sheffield found the misconception in residential homes that 'stroke ... patients are not going to get better, so therapy is not relevant' (Lester, 1994). There is a danger of aphasia going undetected – perhaps being mistaken for the result of hearing loss or dementia – impairments with which care staff will be more familiar. Home managers' expectations will also affect their perceptions of residents' needs for speech and language therapy. Some elderly residents, for example, may be seen as too old and infirm to respond to treatment. This raises questions about the most appropriate input for speech and language therapists. Assessment of individuals' communication impairment and needs is an essential first step. Whilst there are some reports of one-to-one speech and language therapy in residential establishments in Britain (e.g. Bryan and Drew, 1987; Lester, Soord and Trewhitt, 1994), other approaches appear to be favoured. The therapist might work with a group (Bryan and Drew, 1987; Lester, Soord and Trewhitt, 1994), or engage in other strategies to benefit communication-impaired residents. Such strategies include: the provision of advice to care assistants about communicating with particular residents, training for care workers, training of volunteers, initiating and supporting conversation groups run by staff or volunteers, 'befriending' by volunteers and support from a volunteer to enable communication-impaired people to participate in day centre activities. Speech and language therapists must bear the responsibility for initiating such work.

Overall, the evidence suggests a considerable amount of unmet need for speech and language therapy input in residential institutions. Developments in training for care workers are discussed further in Chapters 8 and 9. These developments are to be welcomed, though the extent to which state and private residential homes will invest in such training for their staff is at present unknown. The provision of services to residential homes and to people in residential settings is a new field for many speech and language therapists, and one that requires a different way of working. Therefore opportunities for therapists to develop expertise in working with both staff and residents are called for. In order for this to happen, it is essential that contracts include provision for therapists' clinical development in residential sector work.

SPEECH AND LANGUAGE THERAPISTS WORKING OUTSIDE THE NHS

Some aphasiologists are employed by higher education institutions providing professional education and training in speech and language therapy. Their interests in retaining an active therapeutic role and providing clinical experience for students may be highly compatible with some aphasic people's therapeutic needs. Such institutions are therefore a potential source of aphasia therapy. The long-standing City Dysphasic Group (at City University, London) is an example of therapy located in an academic institution. The group takes referrals from NHS speech and language therapists and is supported by voluntary sector funding.

Purchasing private speech and language therapy is another means of obtaining additional help with language problems. Access does of course depend on the ability to pay; this will exclude many people, especially in view of the loss of income commonly experienced on becoming aphasic (Chapter 2) and the increased costs of disabled living (e.g. Thompson, Buckle and Lavery, 1988). An increasing minority of the British population take out private health insurance. Whilst the amounts paid out will vary from one insurance policy to another, the likelihood is that any cover from private insurance will be insufficient to finance more than short-term aphasia therapy.

Access to private therapy will also be affected by the availability of speech and language therapists outside the NHS. The most comprehensive source of information here is the ADA *National Directory* (1995). Compilation of the material about private provision involved extensive enquiries, including over 200 letters. These elicited, throughout England and Wales, the names of only 30 speech and language therapists who practise privately and take aphasic patients, and three or four additional therapists working in the two partnerships identified. At least a third of these therapists worked part-time in private practice. Private therapists were not spread evenly over the country, with about half living in London and the south-east, and over another third in East Anglia or the West country. None at all were identified in the north of England, the West Midlands or Wales. In general, most private therapists were found in the more affluent parts of the country. ADA's difficulty in obtaining this information makes one wonder how easy it is for aphasic people themselves to access whatever private therapy is available.

Whilst the majority of private therapists worked as sole practitioners in informal settings (their own home or the client's home), a few had their own clinic or a base at a private hospital. Several mentioned that a multi-disciplinary approach was available and a number mentioned referral to other practitioners for occupational or physiotherapy, counselling, music therapy and other 'alternative' therapies. One therapist offered a 'large number of local contacts used to build a programme ... without extra cost to the client' (ADA, 1995, volume 4). The availability of computer software was indicated in some entries. A small number of practitioners had other skills to offer besides speech and language therapy, for example as qualified counsellors and in reflexology and aromatherapy. The largest private speech and language therapy practice included in the volumes of the ADA *Directory* covering England and Wales is in Devon. This comprises the named practitioner and three part-time therapists. This practice has contracts with four fundholding GPs. A sole practitioner in Leicester was the only other private speech and language therapist to mention having entered this market so far. It is not clear from the *Directory* whether these private therapists can offer a specialist aphasia service.

The ADA *Directory* includes a section entitled 'Private rehabilitation'; 15 establishments offering speech and language therapy are listed under this heading. That this is by no means a comprehensive coverage is suggested by indications in a minority of the private speech and language therapists' entries that their work is partly at a private hospital, home or rehabilitation centre. Finance is likely to be the main determinant of access to such facilities as they are very expensive. Fundholding GPs might be a possible source of finance for a minority of patients.

EDUCATION SERVICE PROVISION

Adult education classes are a potential source of language work. Just over half the entries in the ADA *Directory* (1995) indicate some availability to aphasic adults of education service provision. Adult literacy schemes introduced by local education authorities in the 1970s began to attract aphasic 'students', and this led to classes being set up for aphasic people in some areas. Between 1981 and 1983 the Adult Literacy and Basic Skills Unit (ALBSU) funded a project in Essex to develop educational provision for aphasic people. From the start, the need for close co-operation between the speech and language therapy service and adult education was recognized. (Ward and Waugh, 1983, unpublished report). The plan produced by the project envisaged an adult education tutor and a speech therapist working together in adult basic education (ABE) groups for aphasic people, assisted by volunteers and meeting for one morning a week during academic terms.

This scheme has been an additional resource for aphasic people in the areas covered over many years.

The Essex Adult Basic Education scheme shows that it is possible for speech and language therapists and adult education tutors to work together towards a common goal, but it is important to recognize the tensions inherent in such co-operation. Some of the tutor's underlying assumptions may be called into question by the presence of another professional at her class. Similarly, some modification of the speech and language therapist's usual role will be required. Who makes decisions about the programme, for example? A solution used for some time in one group was for the speech and language therapist and tutor to take responsibility for organizing alternate weeks. Another group had little contact with the speech and language therapy service, leaving it without new referrals from speech and language therapists and lacking technical advice, whilst students missed the reassurance of a strong link with speech and language therapy. By 1993, a decision had been made to restrict involvement with the groups in one part of Essex to one visit a term. This withdrawal resulted from a conflict in philosophy between the needs-led NHS and an education service led by student demand. The speech and language therapy manager felt that, to justify more frequent contact, goals should be set for each aphasic person referred, with discharge once the goal was attained. This was unacceptable to the education service, whose view was that any decision to leave the group was for the student to make.

A different pattern for co-operation between health and education services has been established in Worcestershire. The Acquired Brain Injury Unit (formerly Acquired Aphasia Unit) based at Evesham College of Further Education is financed partly by local health authorities and receives referrals from speech and language therapy. It has its own management committee. In the past it employed two coordinators, one a speech and language therapist and the other with a background in education (Molteno and Powell, 1990), but there is no longer any direct speech and language therapy involvement (J. Cooper, 1995, personal communication). Volunteers are recruited to work with aphasic people in their homes. The unit also runs weekly group meetings (attended by aphasic students and some volunteer tutors) in several towns in the area (Molteno and Powell, 1990).

Links between speech and language therapy and education departments may lead to opportunities for some aphasic people to progress to college-based courses. The Bury Speakeasy Club arranged for some of its members to attend an adult education course at a local college of further education. Special training was provided for the course tutors, who were assisted by two Speakeasy volunteers. The participants experienced a different setting, approach and 'ambience' and had the chance to broaden their horizons. Adult education tutors' felt need for access to speech and language therapy expertise is underlined by contacts ADA receives from tutors seeking advice on how to help individual aphasic students who have joined their adult basic education classes.

PROVISION BY VOLUNTARY ORGANIZATIONS

Voluntary organizations are also much involved in provision for aphasic people. The Stroke Association runs by far the largest scheme. In 1995 its Dysphasic Support service was operating in 108 districts in England and Wales. Smaller schemes are run by the Women's Royal Voluntary Service (WRVS) and the British Red Cross Society. From July 1995, however, British Red Cross policy was to concentrate primarily on its core function of responding to emergencies. There are also independent general stroke clubs in some places. These are autonomous, though many are affiliated to The Stroke Association for insurance purposes.

Stroke Association Dysphasic Support provides a weekly group and regular home visits by a volunteer to help aphasic stroke people with their speech and language, also social events and outings. On average each service will have 35–40 volunteers to cover 35–45 patients. The Stroke Association has built up an impressive organizational structure to develop, maintain and nurture its Dysphasic Support. There is a paid, part-time local organizer responsible for each local service. This organizer visits new patients, recruits and inducts volunteers, briefs home visiting volunteers before they meet a new patient, provides continuing support to the volunteers and runs the group. The local organizer is supported by a regional manager who is, in turn, responsible to the director of community services. Recruiting a good local organizer is essential for the success of a service and the speech and language therapy department takes part in the appointment process. Training for new local organizers is provided by the regional manager with input from speech and language therapy and other relevant professionals, and continues during their early months in post.

The development of the service can be seen to some extent as a response to the paucity of speech and language therapy services for stroke patients when it was set up, in 1973, as the Volunteer Stroke Scheme (VSS). At first the VSS seems hardly to have acknowledged the existence of the speech therapy profession, but in recent years better working relationships have developed, in the main. The service is now described by The Stroke Association as 'complementary to the work of the speech and language therapists' (1993a) and the speech and language therapy manager's agreement is sought before a new service is developed. This agreement may or may not be matched by enthusiasm among therapists treating aphasic people. Whilst the vast majority of its referrals come from speech and language therapists, The Stroke Association also accepts referrals from other medical or paramedical sources. Referrals other than from the patient's GP are referred to the GP for advice, and speech and language therapists are informed of referrals not originating from their department (Griffith, n.d.).

Funding arrangements have changed to some extent over the years. Early schemes were funded by the CHSA, with funding being taken over by the local health authority at its discretion. From 1978 the CHSA funded schemes for the initial 2 years only, having obtained prior agreement from the health authority that it would take financial responsibility thereafter, provided the scheme was running successfully. Some schemes have received joint funding from district health authorities and local authority social services for a period, after which they have been health authority funded. More formal contracting arrangements have been introduced under the 1991 NHS reforms (Chapter 6). Some Stroke Association Dysphasic Support services' contracts are with health-commissioning agencies (purchasers), but in many areas Dysphasic Support is now funded via contracts with the NHS trusts responsible for providing speech and language therapy services in the area. This could be seen as symbolizing how integral a part of the service the voluntary provision has become. Since 1993, funding for new Dysphasic Support services has been secured from the outset.

The WRVS runs Speech After Stroke clubs in a number of areas, particularly in the north-east of England. British Red Cross schemes vary to some extent from district to district, for example running a Speech After Stroke club in one city and having several home-visiting volunteers who work closely with a speech and language therapist in a rural area. WRVS schemes co-operate with and receive their referrals from the local speech and language therapy service, but are financially independent. Speech and language therapists' roles in the recruitment of volunteers for such schemes vary.

All the schemes discussed so far are similar in that they provide local, face-to-face services for aphasic people and, to some extent, their carers. In contrast, ADA provides an information and advice service that is used by speech and language therapists, relatives of people with aphasia and others involved in their care, such as nurses, occupational therapists, physio-therapists and adult education tutors. Some 16000 to 20000 booklets in ADA's 'How to Help' series (see Appendix B) are distributed annually. The requirement increasingly being built into NHS contracts for health workers to inform patients about relevant voluntary organizations has led to an increasing demand for literature. ADA's director is a speech and language therapist and other members of the profession are employed for particular projects as funding allows. Speech and language therapists are also involved with ADA in a voluntary capacity, as council and committee members. One of ADA's aims is to increase knowledge and awareness of aphasia, not least at the Department of Health (DoH). The setting up by ADA of local branches is discussed in Chapter 9.

State and voluntary services are often presented as alternatives, as if they are completely discrete means of provision. In practice this is far from being the case (Waine, 1991, Chapter 4). For example, the Stroke Association Dysphasic Support service is funded by the state, through contracts with District Health Authorities (DHAs). Another pattern is for a speech club provided as part of NHS provision to register as a charity, this dual status allowing it to raise funds on its own account and to apply to the government for funding available to charities, and thus to expand its provision for aphasic people without being totally dependent for its resources on NHS contracts.

Our discussion here of the voluntary sector has focused on its role as a direct provider of services. Some of the issues concerning the relationship between voluntary and state provision for aphasic people are considered in subsequent chapters.

APHASIA SERVICES AND MODELS OF DISABILITY

Recipients of health and social services are conceived in the policies described above as relatively passive 'consumers', whose only contribution to the shaping of services lies in the provision of information for evaluation purposes (Chapter 4). Whilst both NHS and community care reforms counted 'consumer choice' among their aims, much evidence suggests that in practice this is most unlikely to be achieved (e.g. Cutler and Waine, 1994). Service provision and service delivery issues tend to be seen as technical rather than political. There is little apparent recognition of social and environmental barriers, let alone strategies for the removal of such barriers as demanded by the disability movement and the social model of disability.

In discussing services we have mainly used the term 'patients', which is probably an accurate reflection of how aphasic people are currently viewed by therapists. British speech and language therapists see their role as being very much concerned with communication in everyday life, rather than merely in the clinic. However, communication difficulties do tend to be seen as the individual impaired person's problem, or as the family's problem. Therapy aims predominantly at enhancing the level of individual aphasic people's communication skills, whilst also paying some attention to their psychosocial well-being. There is clearly a need for a battery of approaches, including those of conventional therapy, and it is important that good practice at an individual level is not devalued in the quest for a broader-based perspective. Some current developments in practice have potential in forwarding a social model approach to aphasia. In particular, the increasing use of contracts opens up the relationship between patient and therapist and will, at best, mean an exchange of information. This will not necessarily be a prelude to therapists relinquishing some power to patients and thus putting their relationship on a more equal footing, but it could be a first step. We know of a few isolated instances in Britain of attempts explicitly to reduce the social barriers created by aphasia, and some are discussed in later chapters.

The final point to make in this chapter is not conducive to academic analysis, or to measured quality standards and the goals of economy, efficiency, effectiveness and value for money that pervade the policy agenda. It is simply to acknowledge the tremendous resource for aphasic people that exists in the expertise of therapists and their commitment to improving aphasic people's quality of life. This is perhaps most evident in the work of the British Aphasiology Society, which is increasingly concerned with the implications of the social model of disability for aphasia services and is taking a lead in promoting new ways of working.

Aphasia services in context

Any service operates within various contexts that together help define and delineate its underlying philosophy and its boundaries. A service will be affected by a wide range of factors, embracing historical, economic, social, geographical, political, ideological, cultural and professional considerations. Such factors may operate at local, national and (increasingly) international levels. The interrelationships between different factors may be complex and are likely to alter over time. Changes in this policy environment will almost certainly impact on service providers, service users and the interaction of front-line staff with their clientele. To understand services fully, we would need to delve into the history of the NHS, speech and language therapy and aphasia services in the UK. Our aim in this chapter is more limited, namely to place aphasia services in their current context in the mid 1990s. We begin the chapter by summarizing recent changes in the organization and management of health care in Britain and identifying some of the implications for speech and language therapy and aphasia services.

Next we locate speech and language therapy in the context of rehabilitation services. We identify some of the structural and attitudinal problems associated with this provision, and discuss the extent to which these are being addressed.

In Chapter 2 our concern was with the impact of aphasia on various facets of people's lives. People's experience, perhaps of a range of service systems, is also relevant to our understanding of the context of aphasia services. We describe briefly the current arrangement of community support services for disabled people.

The contexts outlined above are specific to our society, so much of this chapter pertains, like Chapter 5, to aphasia services in Britain. The final aspect of the service environment certainly has a cultural component, but may nevertheless be more widely applicable. It concerns the needs of people who have suffered a stroke and their responses both to becoming disabled and to the services on offer.

CHANGING HEALTH CARE IN BRITAIN AND APHASIA SERVICES

Speech and language therapy services are provided free at point of delivery on the basis of individual need in Britain as part of NHS provision. They constitute a very small part of the NHS, and policy makers tend to pay them little attention. Under the 1990 NHS and Community Care Act, quasi-markets were created in both health and social care services. Prior to implementation of the health reforms contained in that Act in 1991, District Speech Therapists employed by DHAs had responsibility for meeting the needs of communication-impaired people in their district, in so far as this was possible within the budget allocated to these services. The 1990 Act introduced a quasi-market in health care: a division within the NHS into 'purchaser' and 'provider' structures, thus separating these two roles and creating a contractual basis for the provision of health care, with purchasers specifying the services required and providers in competition with each other for these 'contracts'.[1] Since the 1990 Act the composition of 'purchasers' has changed to some extent. From 1996, purchasers are:

- health-commissioning bodies composed by the merging of the DHA and Family Health Services Authority (FHSA)[2] within each area or consortia covering the geographical area of two or more DHAs/FHSAs, whose responsibility is to assess the health care needs of the district and to ensure that these needs are met;
- fundholding GPs, who are responsible for obtaining certain services for their patients. There are also a number of GP practices taking responsibility for purchasing all health services for their patients as part of Total Purchasing Pilots/Partnerships (TPPs).

Providers consist of:

- family practitioner services;
- NHS hospital and community trusts;
- a small number of units managed directly by the DHA;
- independent sector providers of health services comprising commercial enterprises and voluntary (non-profit) organizations.

These arrangements mean that some GPs act as both purchasers and providers.

The most obvious location for speech and language therapy is with community health services but groupings of services will vary to some extent from area to area.

The NHS is funded mainly through taxation, and operates within financial constraints determined by central government policy (Cutler and Waine, 1994). The introduction of quasi-markets changed the way NHS resources are distributed from national to local level. The pattern of services before the 1991 changes was for the more specialized services to be provided by regional centres located mainly in large cities. DHAs containing regional centres received additional resources to take into account their many patients from other districts.

Since 1991 resources have been channelled through a quango, the NHS Executive, and have then been distributed to all districts on a weighted capitation basis. The per capita funding for a given year is adjusted to take into account the age distribution of a district's population, variations in need and cost differences. Every local health authority is responsible for the health needs of its own population. Through their placing of contracts, health commissioners can now make strategic choices about where to send patients, and this enables established referral patterns to be reassessed and perhaps changed. Some authorities that have traditionally sent patients to specialized facilities outside their areas are developing alternative services nearer home. This may or may not involve a move to community- as against hospital-based services. It does mean that funding for what were formerly regional centres is less secure. The effects of this are most marked in London, with its many long-established hospitals and specialized facilities. The Tomlinson Report (1992) considered the future pattern of health care provision in London and recommended the closure or amalgamation of some hospitals in order to transfer resources into the capital's hitherto underdeveloped primary health services. Anticipated and actual shifts in funding are likely to have consequences for all services, including speech and language therapy.

The 1991 changes were concerned primarily with the delivery of health care to patients, but repercussions for other aspects of the NHS were inevitable. In particular, questions have been raised about future investment in clinical research and professional education under the new system. The CSLT (1993) expressed anxiety about likely detrimental effects on speech and language therapy student placements, research and postgraduate training in its response to the Tomlinson Report.

One consequence of the post-1991 system is a more fragmented pattern of health care organization, making generalization about service provision more difficult than before. There is also far less stability in arrangements, with both purchasers and providers tending to group and regroup to cope with resource constraint and demand problems. We can, however, identify a number of common features. Not all of these are due to the 1991 reforms, though some pre-existing trends have been accentuated by these changes.

The purchaser/provider split shifts the location of decision-making power away from clinical specialists. It is now purchasers who take decisions as to priorities and service development. Main purchasers are very far removed from speech and language therapy, and are most unlikely to be well informed about such a small part of their domain. Thus professional expertise regarding needs may to some extent be devalued. Only services covered by contract can be carried out, so speech and language therapy managers have less freedom to shift resources in response to fluctuating demand. Through the provider hierarchy, service managers must persuade purchasers to provide finance before they can respond to long-standing or newly emerging gaps in provision. Jordan (1994) elicited concern from speech and language therapy managers in two out of three services studied about such inflexibility in the contract-based system. However, the study also reported some evidence of success in getting the case for additional resources accepted and a feeling that speech and language therapy had a stronger voice under the post-1991 system.

Contracting, cost and quality

In a booklet linked to the *Citizens' Charter* initiative (DoH, 1991/1995; Prime Minister's Office, 1991) called simply *Stroke*, the NHS Executive (1995) sets out what stroke patients think are important in the provision of health services. The booklet was intended to inform both purchasers and providers about how to design their stroke services and it effectively conveys statements about stroke services, for instance that patients should be assessed rapidly after the onset of stroke, and that the assessment should be effective and informed. Excerpts from interviews with patients and families illustrate the themes of patient choice and attention to the quality of information for stroke sufferers and their families. One contributor described being spoken about as if she was not present because she could not speak, and another was quoted as saying that he did not want to go to a stroke club because he had seen enough of people being ill. Other sections in the booklet guide purchasers to ask questions of providers such as 'Have you consulted patients and carers about the nature and range of services you are contracting, e.g. through focus groups, The Stroke Association and your Community Health Council?' (p. 20).

Guidance such as the NHS Executive booklet, as well as the inclusion of stroke alongside coronary heart disease as one of the five priority areas targeted by the government in *The Health of the Nation* (DoH, 1992) make it likely that many health purchasers will be drawing up agreements specifically in relation to their local stroke services. There is discussion about the quality of the service specifications and contracts that individual purchasers require. By late 1995 there was still a considerable degree of uncertainty about the standards purchasers would set for stroke services, and hence their implications in terms of pressures on providers. As purchasers operate independently of each other, the strong likelihood is that quality standards will continue to vary from one area to another. Solomon (1995) describes a survey of providers' agreements with purchasers and notes that, whilst there was a high level of concord between purchasers and providers in relation to aspects of services such as access to multi-disciplinary assessment and planned rehabilitation, there was less agreement about purchasers' information requirements for stroke services.

Health commissioners' deliberations about stroke services may mean significant changes in policy, as illustrated by the following example. The main purchaser for stroke services in one English city has stressed the need for integration of acute, rehabilitation and continuing care services, with a shift of emphasis away from treatment of the acute stroke towards rehabilitation and care. The purchaser is also interested in ensuring that voluntary bodies such as The Stroke Association are enabled to participate in providing services in the city and that carers are provided with an opportunity to advise providers and purchasers of their wants and needs. The challenge is to devise a service specification that addresses these recommendations within a given timescale and then to develop a contract that specifies a 'contract currency' that is meaningful. For example, the contract currency might be the number of 'episodes of care'[3] that a district would expect to provide in a year. Meeting that target would ensure only that heads were counted, not that care was appropriate or satisfactory. Perhaps a more sensitive contract currency for stroke might be the number of individual patients who agreed on discharge that their care had met their expectations.

It is worth noting at this juncture the roles of different 'players' in the reformed health care system. There is much interest in researching the needs of consumers and, as shown in the above example and in Chapter 4, service users are increasingly expected to participate in evaluation of services. One of the government's aims was 'to give patients ... greater choice of the services available' (DoH, 1989b). This has not happened (Klein, 1995). The vast majority of secondary health care is, as anticipated by the government (DoH, 1989b), carried out under 'block' or 'cost and volume' contracts rather than 'cost per case' contracts for particular patients (Cutler and Waine, 1994). Therefore money follows the contracts and the patients follow the money. Despite the apparent concern about user involvement, the role of patients in health services is, as suggested in Chapter 4, rather limited. As explained above, the power to make the key decisions about health care provision rests with purchasers. Their decisions, which constrain what is available to a particular patient, may be mediated by a provider such as a non-fundholding GP. It is purchasers, and to some extent providers, rather than the ultimate service users who have 'client power' in the quasi-market system.

Setting and monitoring quality standards are an integral part of service contracting, and should cover aspects of care for aphasia such as the timely sharing of information, a satisfactory discharge from hospital and an acceptable wait for first assessment and treatment. The professional standards document for speech and language therapy *Communicating Quality* (CSLT, 1991) was put together in preparation for contracting. More recently, the British Aphasiology Society has produced a document for purchasers (British Aphasiology Society, 1993), summarizing the issues which should be considered in relation to aphasia. The paper was endorsed by ADA, The Stroke Association and the CSLT and has been distributed to purchasers nationwide, including GP fundholders. It describes the elements of rehabilitation that are relevant to aphasia such as early assessment and advice, and access to counselling services for both patient and carer. It spells out the requirements of a quality service, identifying as important elements the retention of an open referral system and the availability of transport to a rehabilitation centre. Providers who are involved in negotiating service specifications and contracts with purchasers may well find it a useful and authoritative resource that should facilitate the setting of clear, appropriate and realistic contract currencies.

A possible advantage for patients of a contract-based system is that the requirement to fulfil the contract might ensure that cover is provided during staff absence. However, such practice was standard in only one of Jordan's three study areas in 1993. The contracting system increases the administrative burden on services, for example in negotiating contracts and ensuring that new patients are entitled to receive a service (Jordan, 1994). Pound and Sheridan (1994) cite 'increases in administration at the expense of the clinical workload' as one source of stress among therapists working with aphasic and head-injured patients. They found that: 'GP fundholder referrals in particular generated large amounts of paperwork.'

The shift from hospital care and the prioritization of primary care

Many factors have contributed to a shift in emphasis from hospital to primary care and other community-based services. These include technological innovation, demographic trends, changing ideas about best medical practice, patients' preferences and quasi-market forces (Duggan, 1995). In quasi markets, hospitals must provide services as economically as possible in order to tender competitively for contracts. This creates pressure to discharge patients from hospital as early as possible and also leads to reluctance to provide continuing (i.e. long-term) hospital care. The post-1991 changes have been accompanied by re-evaluation of the role of hospitals and of the number of hospital beds required. As noted earlier, this has been most obvious in London, but it has by no means been confined to the capital.

The new and evolving models of health service provision are local and diverse (e.g. Duggan, 1995). Our impression at time of going to press is that the rate of change is, if anything, increasing. Systematic analysis of emerging patterns that may be common to different localities is beyond the scope of this book. We now describe changing institutional patterns in one area by way of illustration. Jordan (1994) found evidence of former long-stay hospitals for elderly people being used for rehabilitation. In the past, these hospitals offered nursing care. During the first half of the 1990s they gradually became more active rehabilitation hospitals as acute units found that they could manage their bed use by moving stroke patients and others into them to vacate beds for 'high tech' services. This meant these hospitals taking selected patients at an earlier stage in their recovery for a much shorter period. The most recent trend in this area has been towards decommissioning of remaining long-stay hospitals, in order to cut estate costs and release monies. The former clientele are now either sent home and offered support there, or enter private nursing homes. Government guidance states that the NHS must provide continuing care where 'the patient needs … ongoing and regular specialist clinical supervision' (DoH, 1995, p. 8). The question of NHS responsibility for continuing care is important to patients for two main reasons. First, they have to make a financial contribution, according to their means, towards the cost of nursing home care provided outside the NHS and for independent or public sector residential care. Second, patients' location may affect their access to rehabilitation services. Our analysis in Chapter 5 of NHS aphasia provision illustrates this last point only too clearly.

To some extent the trends outlined above may limit hospital stay and perhaps lead to major treatment planning decisions being taken at an earlier stage in a patient's recovery from stroke than hitherto, and therefore based on less-reliable predictions of likely outcome. However, because the waiting time for a nursing care place may be relatively long – perhaps 12 weeks or more following referral – the problem may be more apparent than real.

There are national initiatives to move rehabilitation into primary care settings such as local clinics, GP surgeries and clients' homes. The funding previously devoted to long-stay hospitals in the district described above is consequently being directed into rehabilitation services in primary care settings. 'Hospital at Home' and 'Early Discharge' schemes are being developed across the country. The King's Fund has recently initiated a national interest group for schemes such as these, and aims to promote such schemes and to encourage and guide their evaluation of methods of implementation and outcomes for patients. The schemes target a range of client groups, including elderly people and orthopaedic patients. There are also some that focus on stroke.

Even before the 1991 reforms, an Office of Health Economics report (1988) questioned the desirability of hospitalization for stroke patients, suggesting that they do at least as well at home as in hospital. Evidence such as the study by Jordan (1991) suggests that hospitalization is currently the main route giving access to language rehabilitation, and that aphasia is less likely to be referred to speech and language therapy for initial assessment if the patient remains at home. Given the uncertainty about the incidence and prevalence of aphasia (Chapter 3) it is not possible to predict reliably the numbers of aphasic people in particular areas. This means that we cannot estimate 'expected referral rates' so have little firm evidence as to the accessibility of aphasia services. As many as 40% of respondents to the CSLT survey cited without being solicited 'the infrequency of referrals from general practitioners' as a reason for non-referral (Mackenzie *et al.*, 1993, p. 50). Ross (1990) suggests a number of possible reasons for underreferral by GPs, including:

- the small proportion of their patients suffering from speech and language disorders;
- minimal teaching for medical students about speech and language therapy at undergraduate and postgraduate levels;
- the small number of speech and language therapists treating these disorders;
- the fact that these therapists are mainly hospital based.

There appears to be no clear evidence on what effect, if any, GP fundholding is having on referrals of aphasic people for speech and language therapy. Increasing use of primary care settings for therapy may be expected to have some impact here.

The changing pattern of health care has major implications for aphasia services which, historically, have been mainly hospital based. Earlier discharge from hospital after stroke and the reduction in numbers of continuing care beds limit the possibility of speech and language therapy with inpatients, with the therapist's role in some services being limited to one of providing assessment and advice (Pound and Sheridan, 1994), a point we discussed in Chapter 5. For access to speech and language therapy services for aphasic people through the traditional hospital route to be preserved, rapid assessment of communication problems at the acute stage and the availability of a community service are essential. As indicated above, access is likely to be more problematic for stroke patients who are not admitted to hospital. One possible solution might be to seek an outpatient location that is standard for all stroke patients, and to use this as an access route for speech and language therapy. There is pressure from the medical profession for routine CT scanning in stroke diagnosis. This involves attendance at an acute unit, so could offer just such an opportunity. Preliminary screening for speech and language difficulties would need to be built into the neurological assessment to enable referral to speech and language therapy of patients showing any sign of communication impairment. Rehabilitation services need to remain vigilant that traditional routes of access to their services are maintained and that new ones are built in when primary care developments arise.

These trends towards briefer hospital stays and non-hospitalization will also affect the nature of the therapy service required by aphasic people, as they increase the need for outpatient therapy, preferably provided in community settings within easy reach of patients' homes. They will also result in an increase in patients not in hospital who are nevertheless not fit to attend outpatient or community clinics, thus increasing the need for therapy to be provided in patients' homes.

There is an inherent difficulty about developing new systems to ensure that aphasic people are not disadvantaged by the emerging radical changes in health care provision, in that problems of omission – such as missing patients – are by definition hard to detect. The absence of reliable indications of local incidence and prevalence of aphasia is important here. Similarly, it would be all too easy for hard-pressed therapists or services to continue to use selection criteria for treatment that have become less appropriate than they were a few years ago. There must be considerable scope for the sharing of ideas. Particularly because of the culture and nature of the quasi-market system, with its emphasis on competition and fragmented pattern of services, there is a danger that these issues will not be debated at the level necessary for the development of the new policies and practices that are required throughout the country. Therefore the speech and language therapy profession needs urgently to address the shift in provision from acute unit to community in terms of:

- access to services, that is, who will refer to speech and language therapy;
- provision of services, that is, where and how speech and language therapy services will be offered.

The quest to improve cost-effectiveness

Working for Patients, the policy document announcing the NHS reforms (DoH, 1989b) placed a strong emphasis on increasing economy, efficiency, effectiveness and value for money. It followed that great importance was (and is) attached to the measurement of performance in health services. The 1980s had seen attempts to improve management information in the NHS, notably through the collection of a standard set of statistical data (Körner, 1983) and computerization of information systems. In the absence of satisfactory outcome measures, 'patient contacts' and 'episodes of care' have become major performance indicators. Such measures tell us nothing about which patients receive a service, or about the less easily quantifiable dimensions of quality and effectiveness. With the introduction of contracting there was an increased need to collect data not previously considered important, and therefore not resourced. It led to a greater need for clarity about precisely what services offer and about the underlying rationale for this provision. Alongside the emphasis on performance was increased financial stringency. However, speech and language therapy services for adults may have been protected from cuts to some extent in recent years by the anticipated effects of the changes in community care policy fully implemented from 1993 (Jordan, 1994). We outline these changes later in this chapter.

The emphasis on cost-effectiveness in *Working for Patients* (DoH, 1989b) led to discussion about the most productive use of NHS staff, and more specifically about the possibilities of 'skill mix'. The DoH commissioned a study 'to determine the feasibility and effectiveness of using speech and language therapy assistants with different client groups and in different parts of the country' (Davies and van der Gaag, 1993). This study found that 'speech and language therapy assistants undertook a wide range of administrative and clinical tasks' and, whilst districts employing assistants tended to do less well than the control districts on 'throughput' measures (number of new admissions, number of discharges and total number of clients seen), 'speech and language therapists thought that assistants allowed them to see more clients, spend more time planning intervention and less time on administrative tasks, and increased speech and language therapy presence in the settings in which they worked'. Concerns were expressed about 'the time taken to train and supervise [assistants], the added burdens of "thinking for two people", and, in a number of cases, uncertainties about the role of speech and language therapy assistants'. However, clients' and relatives' perceptions of services were 'generally favourable and ... not significantly affected by the introduction of speech and language therapy assistants'. Assistants themselves were generally enthusiastic, despite perceiving the training they received as inadequate, a concern shared by therapists; supervision was also problematic, being described in some cases as minimal and *ad hoc*.

Another aspect of the quest for cost-effectiveness in speech and language therapy concerns changes in the profession's purview and the relative priority to be given to competing demands on therapists' time and expertise. Since the 1980s speech and language therapists in Britain have begun to provide treatment for swallowing difficulties (dysphagia). Stroke is one source of such difficulties, but by no means the only cause. Nearly half the aphasia and head injury therapists who responded to Pound and Sheridan's questionnaire (1994) 'reported pressure to treat dysphagia patients at the expense of others'. Dysphagia appears to be seen as a higher priority than aphasia among doctors (Jordan, 1994; Pound and Sheridan, 1994) possibly because the former can be life threatening and incurs NHS expenditure, since a result of undetected dysphagia is longer hospital stays due to chest infection or malnutrition. Aphasia, in contrast, is no bar to discharge, and aphasia therapy has no readily discernable impact on survival but rather seeks to improve the quality of life. Whilst frustration at being diverted from treating speech and language impairments appears to be the most vociferous reaction among therapists, some identify possible benefits. Dysphagia work raises the profile of speech and language therapists, and renders them an integral and valued part of the multidisciplinary treatment team. This may increase the likelihood of referral for other disorders, creating more opportunities for language assessment and treatment. Also, the therapist is able to identify any aphasia occurring alongside dysphagia.

Health care in Britain has thus seen many changes in recent years, and we can still not anticipate a period of stability in the NHS. There is no systematic evidence as to the effects of this unsettled situation, but we might expect it to take its toll on staff, if not on services.

REHABILITATION SERVICES

Rehabilitation has been defined as 'a process of active change by which a person who has become disabled acquires and uses the knowledge and skills necessary for optimal physical, psychological and social function' (McLellan, 1991, quoting the Disability Committee of the Royal College of Physicians, p. 13). This conceptualizes rehabilitation in terms of change in the disabled person and thus upholds the individual pathology model of disability.

McLellan lists the many professions involved with rehabilitation as: 'medicine (which of course includes surgery), social work, clinical psychology, occupational therapy, physiotherapy, rehabilitation nursing, chiropody, speech therapy, orthotics and prosthetics, rehabilitation engineering, employment training and continuing education' (p. 18). Not all of these services come under the aegis of health services, and a few may span different systems. Occupational therapy, for example, may be offered by the NHS but in recent years increasing numbers of occupational therapists have been employed by local authority social services departments, while medical social workers will be based in a hospital but employed by the local authority social services, so should provide an important link between the hospital and non-NHS community services.

What services individuals are offered after a stroke (in terms of timing, intensity, duration, location and type of service) will depend on many factors including the nature of their impairment, professionals' assessment of their potential for improvement, what is available in their area and local policy and practice. This variability is illustrated by the 'case studies' at the beginning of Chapter 5 (p. 66). Our impression is that NHS stroke rehabilitation services tend to be concentrated mainly in the months following the stroke, with speech and language therapy continuing longer, sometimes for up to 2 years. As far as aphasia itself is concerned, however, there appears to be no time limit on the potential for improvement; someone receiving speech and language therapy to address a specific problem many months or even years after onset can make significant improvements (Jones, 1986; Brindley *et al.*, 1989).

Rehabilitation services are criticized for fragmentation in the sense that each service treats only certain aspects of a disabled person's impairment rather than the whole person (Beardshaw, 1988). This means that the disabled person may receive concurrent treatment from a number of different specialists, something that might or might not be welcome from the recipient's point of view. Problems may be avoided to some extent by coordination among therapists. There is also a need for someone to take responsibility for ongoing monitoring of the impact of services as a whole on the disabled person's quality of life.

'Key worker' schemes represent one attempt to offer a more holistic approach. The key worker has to be someone who is already providing a service that involves regular contact with the disabled person, whose role is 'to coordinate an individual plan and provide education and positive support' (King's Fund Forum on Stroke, 1988). It is important that role boundaries are clearly identified and that all concerned (including the disabled person) know what they are. Otherwise there is much scope for misunderstanding. Critics of this approach point out that role conflicts may arise for the key worker.

'Case management' is another approach, imported into Britain from the USA. A case management approach avoids the dual role difficulty because the case manager's sole job is to help disabled people negotiate the service system and, where appropriate, act as their advocates or support their self-advocacy. The 1980s saw a number of experimental case management projects in health and social care settings in Britain (Hunter, 1988). One disadvantage is that case management introduces yet another tier of professionals. Large-scale implementation of case management in the public sector, most notably as 'care management' in community care policy (as explored in the next section), has had the effect of changing its focus from advocacy to rationing.

For either type of scheme to work to its full potential, the key worker or case manager will need some knowledge about the possible contribution and local availability of the whole range of rehabilitation services. This could probably be provided most efficiently and effectively by disabled people themselves, but their employment for such purposes is an unknown entity. Jordan (1991) found some evidence of speech and language therapy input in nursing courses, and a therapist giving talks to other remedial therapists and social workers. Similarly, other professions have much to contribute to the training of speech and language therapists. It is not clear whether the necessity in the reformed NHS for a contract and interservice payment for such work acts as a deterrent. Voluntary organizations employing rehabilitation professionals may contribute to interprofessional education through input to professional journals and meetings and by giving specialist advice to practitioners regarding individuals in their care. There has been limited experimentation, in a small number of educational institutions, with courses for the remedial therapies involving some joint teaching for undergraduates. The DoH has accepted a need for 'university-based faculties of health science in which all the [rehabilitation] professions can learn together' and 'a critical mass of academic staff in clinical academic environments to undertake much needed research' (McLellan, 1991, p. 20). This statement appears to assume, however, that the study of disability and rehabilitation are primarily about health – a proposition that is, of course, rejected by proponents of the social model of disability.

A more radical idea would be to combine the three therapy occupations into a single remedial profession. Restructuring of remedial therapy is more than a theoretical possibility, as shown by recent work to design training for a new breed of 'generic health care worker' (Eastwood and Thompson, 1995). It is not clear to what extent such workers would be expected to replace existing specialist occupations, but presumably one attraction for policy makers would be anticipated savings in cost. In our view, 'repackaging' of the therapy professions in any major way would be likely to lead to deskilling, poorer-quality services, new forms of fragmentation and staff demoralization. As we saw in Chapter 4, aphasia therapy requires a great deal of technical knowledge and skill. Initial thinking about generic health care worker training appears to be seriously flawed, making the false assumption that 'standards in common' can be prescribed in relation to practices common to different health care professions, such as 'taking case histories, offering counselling, enabling clients to develop skills and knowledge about their own treatment and helping them to access other services' (Eastwood and Thompson, 1995). As Eastwood and Thompson point out, 'the similarity of these activities among the different professions is spurious', because the *content* and *use* of, for example, a case history are very different. French expresses concern that persuading health and welfare personnel to treat the person (rather than only treating the disorder) may serve to give professionals control over more aspects of disabled people's lives (1994b).

Our evidence suggests that speech and language therapists do often work closely with the other remedial professions, especially physiotherapy, in relation to particular aphasic people. Services can be set up in such a way as to facilitate contact, and thereby the development of mutual trust and respect for other professionals' expertise. An example here is the attachment of teams of remedial therapists to GP practices.

Silburn (1994) describes the work of the integrated living team in North Derbyshire, which uses a social model approach to rehabilitation. The team comprises a coordinator, an occupational therapist, a physiotherapist and a speech and language therapist. The team adopts a key worker approach, and therapists work across specialisms. They 'use each other's professional expertise ... and from time to time conduct joint visits if specialist assessments are needed' (p. 252). To the discomfort of health service staff in other areas, team members have gradually tried to drop their original professional titles. Presumably the integrated living team can enable disabled people to access specialist services, such as aphasia therapy, and here the team's professional knowledge will no doubt ensure that referrals are made and that they are appropriate.

Beardshaw (1988) identified many other problems in rehabilitation, including:

- low priority within the NHS – a general lack of medical interest in 'low-tech', non-curative medicine coupled with conflicting views on whether rehabilitation should be a separate specialism in its own right, a service for other consultants, or a direct and ongoing concern of all specialties;
- attitudes of some professionals that obstruct the development of 'partnership' with disabled people;
- underdevelopment of community remedial therapy owing to chronic staff shortages;
- development of remedial services without reference to the other services that are important for people with disabilities, namely institutional care and community support services;
- poor coordination between hospital and community medicine, with role confusion here leading sometimes to conflicting advice, or to GPs taking little interest;
- lack of effective follow-up in the community from specialist rehabilitation units, due often to the distance between a unit and the disabled person's home;
- absence of coordination between NHS, local authority and voluntary services;
- wide variations in provision between different parts of the country, because development has depended largely on the enthusiasm of individual doctors.

She concludes that: 'there is presently nothing approaching a comprehensive network of rehabilitation services at national, regional or local level' and that there is: 'particular concern about the inadequate services currently available for people with neurological disorders ... [which] reflects a level of disquiet with the traditional role of neurology, and its heavy emphasis on diagnosis' (pp. 20–1).

In our view these criticisms are still relevant in the mid 1990s. The NHS reforms focused on medical and nursing care and paid little attention to rehabilitation services (Rooney, 1989; Turner, 1989). There are some signs of change, however. Rehabilitation medicine was classified by the DoH as a separate specialty in 1989 (McLellan, 1991).[4] Our discussion earlier in this chapter suggests that health commissioners are beginning to challenge at least some of the shibboleths concerning NHS priorities and provision. The government's insistence that local authorities and health services should have joint procedures for hospital discharge may have had some impact on this one aspect of coordination. However, increasingly tight constraints on spending coupled with expanding needs due to the changing health care practices discussed above and a reduction by the NHS in the responsibility it takes for continuing care are eroding the ability of many social services departments to deliver community care services (Age Concern London, 1995; Association of County Councils/Association of Metropolitan Authorities, 1995).

COMMUNITY SUPPORT SERVICES FOR DISABLED PEOPLE

We have already begun to consider community support services within the framework of rehabilitation. Organizationally, however, they are composed of a number of quite separate services, with their own distinct sets of mores, rules and regulations, and this is how they appear from the disabled person's perspective. We discussed the role in relation to aphasic people of NHS aphasia services, the voluntary sector and education services in Chapter 5. Here we focus on social security, employment services and local authority social services.

Social security

Many aphasic people are dependent on state benefits. The state social security system in Britain provides benefits to cover periods of illness and incapacity for work. There are also benefits to assist with the additional costs of disabled living, and a benefit to top up low earnings for certain disabled people returning to work. Other benefits include retirement pensions, a means-tested safety net and financial assistance for low-income primary carers of some severely disabled people. The system is extremely complicated and entitlement to specific benefits depends on meeting detailed eligibility criteria. The social security system as a whole constitutes by far the largest social welfare programme in terms of expenditure (Hills, 1993), and limiting this expenditure is a major concern of governments. The number of benefits and sheer complexity of the system might lead to the false impression that disabled people's income needs are well catered for (Barnes, 1991). However, criticisms of the system include inadequate levels of benefits in relation to needs, inequity among different groups of disabled people, confusion of 'disability' with 'illness' in the way benefits are constructed, disincentives for disabled people to enter employment, the system's underlying assumptions of individual pathology of disability, and detrimental effects for people dependant on welfare – in particular 'a systematic erosion of personal autonomy and excessive bureaucratic regulation and control' (Barnes, 1991, p. 121; Disability Alliance, 1995; Gibbs, 1995). Where benefits depend on assessments of functional incapacity there is a danger that disability stemming from 'invisible' and poorly understood disorders like aphasia may be underestimated, putting those concerned at a disadvantage as claimants. Jordan (1995a) describes different ways in which disability is assessed within the benefits system and discusses the possible roles of speech and language therapists, such as referral to the Benefits Agency or to other agencies that give benefits information and advice, facilitating communication between a benefits adviser or the Benefits Agency and the communication-impaired person, and providing claimants with supporting evidence.

Employment

Factors with some bearing on aphasic people's employability include general labour market trends, employment and training services and possible antidiscrimination legislation. Recent years have seen a major restructuring of the British labour market, with a shift from manufacturing to service industries, and long-term, mass unemployment continuing alongside a growth in low-paid, part-time jobs. Attempts by both private and public sector employers to minimize costs has also led to a decrease in job security at all levels (Hutton, 1995, p. 224).

Employment services include assistance in finding employment, incentives for employers who take on a disabled person, help with the costs of special equipment, adaptations to the workplace and transport or a support worker to enable a disabled person to work, rehabilitation courses and supported employment. Some aphasic people might qualify for a work training scheme (Disability Alliance, 1995).

Since the beginning of the 1980s there have been many attempts by members of parliament to introduce bills to outlaw discrimination against disabled people. In 1994 the government accepted the case for legislation. The limited measures included in the 1995 Disability Discrimination Act fall short of the civil rights approach taken in some other countries (for example, in New Zealand, Canada, Australia and the USA) (Royal Association for Disability and Rehabilitation (RADAR), 1994) and called for by the disability movement in Britain (e.g. Bynoe, Oliver and Barnes, 1991). The Act makes it unlawful for an employer with 20 or more employees 'to treat a disabled person less favourably because of their disability, without justifiable reason' (Minister for Disabled People, 1995, p. 5). A disabled person is one whose disability is 'substantial' in the employment context and this will include many aphasic people. Employers are expected to make 'reasonable adjustments', for example by recasting job descriptions, altering hours of work, arranging training and providing or modifying equipment. That the Act holds potential benefits for aphasic people is clear, but what is required of employers remains less so. This is because precise meanings of terms like 'substantial disability', 'justifiable reason' and 'reasonable adjustment' will emerge only through regulations, codes of practice and case law once the legislation is in force. We know little about employers' attitudes towards communication-impaired people; these are particularly important since large numbers of small employers are not subject to the legislation.[5] One prediction is that the Act will follow experience in the USA and, rather than assisting unemployed disabled people to get a job, will mainly help people already in work to retain their employment after becoming disabled (Paton, 1995).

Local authority social services

Anderson (1992) suggests that 'social services and social workers should participate more as sources of advice about and for other services' and that: 'As such, these services should be at the heart of a comprehensive policy for longer-term support after stroke" (p. 231). Since the implementation in 1993 of the community care provisions in the 1990 NHS and Community Care Act, local authority social services have had a duty to assess elderly and disabled people's needs for community care services and for state-assisted residential care.[6] 'Care managers' employed by the social services department are responsible for carrying out the assessments and, where it is judged necessary, for putting together 'care packages' tailored to the needs and preferences of each individual,[7] in so far as this is possible within their budgets (Griffiths, 1988; DoH, 1989a). Services may include technical aids, adaptations to the disabled person's accommodation, home care and a range of services to improve the disabled person's quality of life. The intention is that local authority social services departments should act as enabling authorities, rather than being the sole providers. This means contracting independent sector organizations – both voluntary (non-profit-making) bodies and commercial enterprises – to provide some services. In the absence of existing independent providers, local authorities are expected to stimulate their development. Where home adaptations are required to enable the disabled person to stay at home or existing accommodation is judged unsuitable, the local housing authority or a housing association may also be involved.

Beardshaw's (1988) powerful critique of all community services for people with physical disabilities shows the severe limitations of these services and how unsatisfactory they can be from the disabled person's point of view. In particular, provisions for people with continuing disabilities have been beset by problems of insufficient or inappropriate provision and lack of coordination between (and in some instances within) the wide range of agencies involved.

The 1993 community care changes were only to some extent an attempt to tackle these problems. Boundaries between some services are unclear and shifting, in particular between the NHS and local authority social services (Nocon, 1994). This is of significance to disabled people because, as explained earlier, public sector health services in Britain are free at point of delivery, whilst charges may be (and increasingly are) made for local authority domiciliary and day care services. These charges must be 'reasonable' but within this constraint are determined by each local social services authority. Resourcing remains a central issue; many local authorities have withdrawn altogether from assistance with domestic tasks such as cleaning, replacing 'home helps' by 'home care' services to provide personal assistance to more severely disabled people. It is recognized (DoH, 1989a) that informal care – from the disabled person's family and, perhaps, friends and neighbours – accounts for the greatest volume of community support. The 1995 Carers (Recognition and Services) Act gives carers the right to a separate assessment of their needs by the local authority. Implementation of this Act in 1996 without any anticipation of additional funding can only add to the pressure on local authority social services resources.

A minority of aphasic people, albeit a substantial number,[8] live in long-stay institutions. Studies of communication impairment among older people in nursing homes (Jordan *et al.*, 1993) and residential care (Gravell, 1988; Bryan and Drew, 1989; Lendrem and Hurst, 1990) suggest that a small percentage of residents in a particular institution are likely to be aphasic following stroke illness and that these will form a minority of the communication-impaired residents. None of these studies reflects recent experience in Britain where community care policy, especially since 1993, may well lead to a greater concentration of severely disabled people in residential care. This is because only people for whom the cost of support in their own homes exceeds that of residential care will have access to state-assisted residential care.

APHASIC PEOPLE'S NEEDS AND RESPONSES

Earlier chapters include much discussion about aphasic people's needs in relation to communication. Here we draw on the insights of medical sociology for interpretation of disabled people's needs and relationship with services at different points in their 'careers'[9] as disabled people. Bury (1991) considers the nature of individual responses to chronic illness. He draws on sociological studies of a wide range of conditions but not, unfortunately, stroke. Nevertheless, his perceptions add another dimension to any analysis of people's needs following stroke. Whilst Bury is concerned with chronic illness, the concepts can be applied equally in relation to acquired disability.

Bury's conceptualization of the onset of illness as a 'biographical disruption' fits particularly well with the suddenness and unexpectedness that characterizes stroke illness. Bury distinguishes between two types of 'meaning' in chronic illness: its **consequences** and its **significance**. In Chapter 2 we considered consequences of being aphasic following a stroke in relation to communication, income, employment, mobility, everyday activities, leisure and family life. We discussed its significance in terms of people's feelings about being aphasic and their self-perceptions.

As soon as they are well enough, people who have just suffered a stroke will begin to consider the 'longer-term implications of their altered circumstances' (Bury, 1991, p. 455). Bury argues that initially one of the main concerns is to find a meaningful explanation for what has happened, in order to establish some degree of control over their condition. Ireland (Ireland and Black,1992) expresses this very vividly:

> Later, lots of questions for me. Why I could not follow talking? Why I could follow rhythms but not words of songs on the radio? Why I knew to speak only short words? Why not able to read newspapers and books? Why I draw but not write sentences? Why to print and not to use my handwriting? I had to fight this ordeal with truth.
>
> (p. 356)

Bury (1992) shows that people often search out medical and other information about the illness, its causes and prognosis, whilst Anderson (1992) lists the explicit areas of knowledge sought by stroke patients and their carers: 'causation of the stroke and risk of recurrence; prognosis and rate of recovery; mental health and social isolation; services available and what they can do to help themselves' (p. 223). Obtaining information is likely to be difficult for aphasic people early on, owing to the very nature of the impairment. ADA's production of a booklet (1990) giving a simple visual explanation of stroke and aphasia can be seen as an attempt to begin to address this need. Carers and other 'significant others' may take on the task of seeking information, perhaps contacting ADA or The Stroke Association, or both. As implied above, carers are unlikely to be acting simply as agents for the aphasic person here: one group saw information as their priority need, above support and respite care.

The other need at first is for **legitimation**, 'the process of attempting to repair disruption, and establish an acceptable and legitimate place for the condition within the person's life' (Bury, 1991, p. 456). A person whose aphasia was initially misdiagnosed as being due to a mental health problem was relieved at the diagnosis of stroke, which was in tune with her own belief that her inability to speak had a physical cause. The diagnosis here represented, in Bury's words, 'an official validation of the condition' (p. 456). Legitimation is difficult if the disabled person's perceptions and goals clash with those of others. Differences of interpretation may occur in health care settings as well as in everyday life. Widespread ignorance of aphasia, coupled with its invisibility, makes it very likely that aphasic people will have to cope with perceptions that conflict with their own. Defining conflicting positions as resulting from other people's ignorance might help aphasic people to disregard them. We address the issue of how to tackle such ignorance in Chapter 9.

Legitimation may re-emerge as a problem at a later stage, for example owing to consequences either of the condition or of treatment that are considered minor by health professionals but that are important to the disabled person. An example would be the difficulty experienced by an aphasic person in using a communication aid in a particular setting or relationship. Furthermore, as Bury (1991) points out: 'A new "crisis of credibility" may occur if the individual continues to report problems after their "share" of attention has been used up, or when they have been placed in a category ... which closes off avenues of support and information' (p. 457). For some aphasic people, such a crisis might occur when active speech and language therapy comes to an end. As we have seen, many speech and language therapy managers are very aware of the need for 'after-care' services, though there will not always be anything suitable available for particular aphasic people or in a given locality.

The treatment regimen itself also has an impact on patients. Of particular relevance in the context of aphasia services is the 'work' required of patients. It is clear that attention needs to be paid to how this fits in with the person's life, and whether conflicts arise that might affect the patient's compliance. For instance, a person's previous experience of the education system might affect how they feel about doing language exercises, perhaps of a very basic nature, as 'homework'. It might not be obvious that there was a problem to be addressed here, even during negotiation between therapist and patient as to the treatment 'contract'. Bury's analysis (1991) tends to validate contracting. He suggests that: 'Negotiating over the appropriate use and effects of treatment regimens as well as the significance of symptoms enhances adaptation to a disrupted biography' (p. 460).

The importance of emotional aspects of disability should not be underestimated. The need for emotional support may be more generally accepted early on than at a later date. Emotional needs continue to change for a long time post-stroke; they may become more, rather than less, intense as time passes (Kagan and Gailey, 1993), or change in nature. It is often assumed that people 'come to terms' with disability, but some evidence suggests that many people do not (e.g. Parr, 1994). Mildly aphasic people's emotional support needs are at least as great as those of the more seriously impaired (Kagan and Gailey, 1993). Bury (1991) identifies the nature of 'support' as 'the ability to confide in others' (p. 462), indicating the importance of language and communication in access to help from other people.

Endnotes

[1]Contracts with NHS providers deviate from the technical meaning of the term in that there is no recourse to law in the event of alleged breach of conditions. The alternative term 'service agreements' may also be used.

[2]The bodies responsible until 1996 for managing family practitioner services, which include GP services, dentists, pharmacists and opticians.

[3]An 'episode of care' would be defined here as the totality of NHS provision from an individual's entry into the health care system for a particular health problem and his or her discharge from NHS services. The same concept might also be used in relation to a specific service such as speech and language therapy.

[4]In Scotland rehabilitation medicine has been a recognized specialty since 1975.

[5]The exemption of firms employing fewer than 20 staff is to be reviewed after 5 years.

[6]State-assisted residential care includes places in local authority residential homes and means-tested financial assistance with the cost of residential or nursing home care in the local authority or independent sector. The 1990 NHS and Community Care Act gives local authorities a financial incentive to rely on independent sector provision.

[7]At time of going to press, the 1996 Community Care (Direct Payments) Bill was before parliament. This provides for local authorities to make payments directly to disabled people so that they can purchase their own community support services.

[8]The latest official survey of disabled people in Great Britain (Martin, Meltzer and Elliot, 1988) estimates that 422 000 disabled people live in communal establishments. Of a sample of residents in such establishments, 14% were stroke sufferers and just over half of these people had a communication disability (Martin, White and Meltzer, 1989). This would give a 'guesstimate' of just under 30 000 communication-impaired stroke people in communal establishments. Not all of these people will be aphasic, however.

[9]In sociology the concept of 'career' is sometimes used to denote patterns of experience over a period of time.

The volunteer contribution | 7

Volunteers are increasingly involved with aphasic people, providing social support and sometimes assisting more directly with language-related work. Their involvement raises a number of questions, particularly about the respective roles of speech and language therapists and volunteers, about possible implications for the speech and language therapy profession, and about communication between therapists, volunteers, clients and, in some instances, volunteer organizers.

As the CSLT (1991) states: 'The use of volunteers has been well documented in the speech and language therapy literature.' More specifically, there have been a number of studies over many years of voluntary work with aphasic people. Griffith described the pioneering work of the CHSA Volunteer Stroke Scheme[1] (Griffith, 1975, 1980; Griffith and Miller, 1980). Lesser and Watt's evaluation of the Speech After Stroke project in Newcastle upon Tyne suggested that the benefits of a club are 'social rather than linguistic' (1978, p. 1047). A recent study of Stroke Association Dysphasic Support in Leeds (Geddes, Poulter and Chamberlain, 1995) confirms the social benefits. Geddes and colleagues also found some evidence of improved communication ability, but the small number of subjects and absence of any control group here mean that this finding must be treated with caution.

Other studies have tended to concentrate on the comparative efficacy of volunteers and speech therapists. One compared patients receiving speech therapy as outpatients between three and fives times a week, including a group session when possible, with patients who received four home visits a week from volunteers and attended a group session (Meikle *et al.*, 1979). Outcomes were similar for the two kinds of treatment. Another study compared patients who received 2 hours speech therapy a week with others who had 2 hours 'therapy' from untrained volunteers, and also found little difference in recovery between the two groups. They concluded that 'a large part of the improvement ... is the result of the interest, support, and stimulation provided by speech therapist and volunteer alike' (David, Enderby and Bainton, 1982, p. 96).

Wade has emphasized the considerable expenditure of speech therapy time that may be entailed in providing a volunteer service. (Wade, 1983). In both the comparative studies cited above speech therapists recruited volunteers, provided them with some basic information about the nature of stroke and aphasia, matched volunteers with patients and gave general support. Volunteers' work was guided by the speech therapist's assessment and advice, which may well have been crucial to the volunteers' success.

One study that compared costs of volunteer involvement and speech therapy (Quinteros et al., 1984) found that a community speech therapy programme comprising monthly speech therapy at home, a monthly visit for speech practice from a volunteer and a fortnightly group speech therapy session attended also by volunteers incurred greater costs to the speech therapy department than monthly outpatient appointments. Fortnightly or weekly outpatient speech therapy was, however, more expensive than the community speech therapy programme. Also, patients allocated to the latter were assessed as having improved more than the outpatients. The community speech therapy patients received considerably more attention than the outpatients, especially as their attendance at group sessions was higher than the outpatients' attendance for speech therapy. A factor that may have affected attendance was that the volunteers provided transport for the community speech therapy patients.

These studies were all based on different treatment regimens, and all involved comparatively small numbers of aphasic people. They give no information about the specific speech therapy techniques used by the therapists, or about the nature of the practice provided by the volunteers. They are also not without methodological difficulties (David, Enderby and Bainton, 1983; Meikle and Wechsler, 1983; Pring, 1983); in particular the practice of comparing groups of patients is questionable, given the complexity of aphasia, and in one study (David, Enderby and Bainton, 1983a) assessment was problematic. We must therefore be wary of generalizing from these studies. They do show, however, that volunteer involvement can be helpful, and give some indication of the costs that may be incurred.

The above literature construes volunteer involvement as a means to assist in the management of aphasia and the amelioration of its effects by 'treating' individual aphasic people. It thus reflects the individual model of disability. Wertz (1989) argues for what he calls an 'ecological' approach to therapy, concerned with 'how aphasic patients relate to their environments', and envisages asking volunteers 'to administer treatment designed to assist aphasic people in doing what they did before becoming aphasic ... in patients' homes' (p. 9). He goes on to suggest that therapists should design treatment to accomplish aphasic people's own goals. This has some elements of social model thinking. Social model ideas may be evident in the attitudes and actions of some volunteers, even within quite traditional schemes, and also in the philosophy of some schemes. The words and actions of other volunteers working to an individual pathology, 'personal tragedy' model of disability within the latter would lead to a significant divergence between theory and practice and, in effect, a negation of a scheme's social model stance.

We know that volunteers participate in aphasia services in many parts of Britain. A survey conducted in the mid 1980s found that two-thirds of the 76 health districts that responded involved volunteers, who in 48% of these were deployed with stroke/aphasic people (Speech Therapy in Practice, 1987). Exactly the same percentage of districts reported using volunteers with aphasic people to the CSLT Aphasia Working Party national survey carried out in late 1990 (Mackenzie *et al.*, 1993). The number of services with volunteers may have increased during the 1990s, not least due to the continuing expansion of the Stroke Association Community Services, Dysphasic Support scheme. Three-quarters of the 211 services in England and Wales submitting information for the ADA *National Directory* (1995) indicated some current use of volunteers. (The use of this directory as a source is discussed in Chapter 5.) Volunteers may be 'employed' to work with aphasic people by:

- NHS speech and language therapists;
- other public sector bodies, notably local education departments;
- voluntary organizations.

Of the voluntary organizations, as noted in Chapter 5 The Stroke Association runs by far the largest service in Britain. During 1994 this service in England and Wales 'employed' 3813 volunteers and helped 5616 stroke people. Analogous schemes are run by the CHSAs, in Scotland and Northern Ireland. The Stroke Association model is now established in a number of countries, including Australia, New Zealand and the Republic of Ireland. In Chapter 5 we described the Stroke Association Dysphasic Support service and the smaller schemes run in Britain by the WRVS and the British Red Cross Society.

In the following sections of this chapter, we first consider who volunteers and why. We then examine the case against volunteer involvement, before exploring the nature of the volunteers' work. We identify some parameters for successful voluntary work with aphasic people and focus on training as a key issue here. We discuss the need for guidelines for speech and language therapists to good practice on volunteer involvement. Finally we describe a project based on the ideas of the social model of disability to illustrate how volunteers can work within such a context.

WHO ARE THE VOLUNTEERS?

Voluntary work is sometimes assumed to be a female, middle class and middle-aged occupation. The 1992 *General Household Survey* (Goddard, 1994) found limited support for this stereotype. Respondents were asked about their participation in voluntary work over the previous year. Women's participation rates were higher than men's, but not dramatically so. Also, people in paid work were more likely than the unemployed or economically inactive, to have been involved in voluntary work, women in part-time employment being the most active group. Professional people were several times more likely to have been engaged in voluntary work than unskilled workers. The peak age for voluntary work was 35–44 years, followed closely by 45–59 years. There were some differences between the sexes in the types of activity undertaken, with men being more likely to serve on management committees, for example.

Evidence on the characteristics of volunteers who work with aphasic people is patchy and fragmented. The Stroke Association Dysphasic Support volunteers span a very wide age range, from college students to retired people. The latter, probably the largest group, include some people who have taken early retirement. Some volunteers have themselves recovered from stroke (M. Miles, 1995, personal communication). In Leeds, the single largest group of volunteers (a third of the 28) 'described themselves as homemakers' (Geddes, Poulter and Chamberlain, 1995). Most were in their 40s and 50s. The wide range of occupations and former occupations of volunteers is illustrated by the list from the Leeds study: 'nurses, secretaries, bank staff, a company director, office workers, a hairdresser, a clergyman, a pharmacy technician, domestic workers, a teacher, a lecturer and a student' (p. 10). The most striking feature of this group of volunteers was the sex ratio of 24 women to 4 men. Of about 3800 volunteers working in Stroke Association Dysphasic Support in 1994, just under 80% were women.

Information was obtained by Jordan (1990, 1991 and unpublished data) on some 15 clubs and schemes involving volunteers with aphasic people. These included groups and clubs run with the assistance of volunteers by speech and language therapists, adult basic education clubs for aphasic people, a scheme employing volunteers to encourage the use of communication aids and two (then) VSSs. Whilst the sex ratios varied among these clubs and projects, women predominated as volunteers in every one. A partial explanation for this might be that daytime services are needed because of the fatigue that often accompanies aphasia and this excludes more men than women as volunteers. Men who volunteered often did so initially as drivers for a group, and might later be drawn into working within the group as well.

In most schemes, volunteers tended to be middle aged or older. Other clusters of volunteers were women with family responsibilities and disabled people. Two projects were funded by a government scheme (Opportunities for Volunteering) to enable unemployed people to gain experience as volunteers. Not surprisingly, these projects recruited volunteers with a younger age profile (e.g. Purdy, 1985).

A few volunteers' interest had been kindled by the experience of a relative who had suffered a stroke or head injury. One had himself been aphasic due to a war injury from which he had fully recovered many years before. Several speech and language therapists commented that the line between 'helper' and 'helped' is a blurred one. There are several aspects to this observation:

- The intended recipients of the service may help each other.
- Recent 'recipients' might become volunteers.
- Some recipients and volunteers have characteristics in common, such as age and/or disability. A few volunteers had speech impairments, such as a stammer, or difficulties resulting from a progressive disease like multiple sclerosis, or other physical impairments. A few more had suffered nervous breakdowns.[2]
- Volunteers themselves have needs that they are attempting to meet by volunteering (Moore, 1985). The regular commitment helped to give structure and purpose to the day for people who were unemployed, retired or out of the labour market owing to family commitments or disability. There might also be practical benefits. Examples here include, for unemployed people, gaining experience that might improve their chances of securing employment and, for a volunteer with a stammer, speech practice in a sheltered environment.

Becoming a volunteer was a way of making a contribution to society. More specific reasons were concern about standards of literacy (an ex-adult literacy volunteer) and preferring to undertake daytime voluntary work. One Stroke Association service found that over half its volunteers had prior experience of stroke, either through their work or through personal contact with a stroke person (Geddes, Poulter and Chamberlain, 1995). Our impression, however, was that relatively few volunteers had any knowledge of aphasia before being recruited to their particular scheme.

The attraction for volunteers of work with aphasic people has been described as follows by the founder of the VSS:

- [Volunteers] are being offered constructive, positive work that will exercise their minds and ingenuity, and give scope to their goodwill ... they are given information, advice and guidance, and positive ways of helping the patient are suggested, but they are also free to use their own ideas, interests and personality.

- They will be working *directly with* the person who needs help, and not middle-men in the chain of committee, administration or money-raising efforts.

(Griffith, n.d., p. 5)

THE CASE AGAINST VOLUNTEERS

The Quirk Report registered the committee's:

conviction that there is in the work of the speech therapist an element, partly consisting of ancillary work but including some aspects of treatment, which is routine and repetitive and does not call for the skill and knowledge of a speech therapist.

(Department of Education and Science, 1972, p. 83)

Some members of the Quirk committee 'had had experience of the successful use of voluntary workers ... under the supervision of a speech therapist' (ibid., p. 84). Despite this, it was not to volunteers that Quirk looked to fulfil tasks that speech therapists might delegate, but to paid speech therapy aides. Whilst some speech therapy aides have been appointed, their numbers have never been large. The increasing involvement of volunteers must therefore be seen in the context of health authorities' failure, for whatever reasons, to implement Quirk's recommendations regarding aides (now termed assistants).

There is no consensus among speech and language therapists regarding volunteers. Opposition centres round a number of issues, including ethics, the state of aphasia therapy, resource implications and negative impact on the therapy profession.

Ethics

A distinction is made between relatives, for whom helping a member of their family to overcome aphasia is part of an ongoing relationship, and volunteers, who do not have such a bond. Foggitt (1987) has argued that speech and language therapists 'have a relationship of confidence, trust and privacy with ... patients, and involving people who have no similar bond is wrong and unprofessional' (p. 29). Speech and language therapists could be justified in using volunteers if they could retain complete control of them, but the close supervision and monitoring that would be required to do this are not possible. As many as 18% of the districts using volunteers who responded to the national survey of Mackenzie *et al.* (1993) admitted involving volunteers in therapy not directed by a speech and language therapist. This would seem to be incompatible with professional standards of accountability and outcome evaluation, as stated in *Communicating*

Quality (CSLT, 1991). Another issue concerns confidentiality, and the risk that this will be breached. Foggitt (1987) suggests that, whether or not this happens 'the fear that trust will be betrayed is a real and destructive one' (p. 29). It is also held that people have a right to expect and to receive treatment by professionals in the NHS.

The state of aphasia therapy

Aphasia therapy has been developing very rapidly over the last decade, and therapists should therefore have more to offer in the way of therapy to address a particular patient's impairment specifically than at the time of the 'group trials' discussed at the beginning of this chapter. Volunteers, however well trained and committed, do not have the expertise to replace the speech and language therapist, and should not be put in the position of being expected to do so by becoming responsible for providing the only service someone gets too soon after their stroke. Furthermore, by limiting the contact they have with patients, working through volunteers gives speech and language therapists less opportunity to reach the in-depth understanding of patients' language problems that is required to make progress in devising more effective treatment strategies. Volunteer involvement is therefore likely to retard the development of more effective therapy.

Resource implications

One argument here is about the cost:benefit ratio. The more resources put into careful selection and training of volunteers the less time is saved by speech and language therapists. If volunteers' performance were properly monitored, they would become even more expensive in terms of therapists' time. In the past these costs were often 'hidden' since they did not appear as separate items in speech therapy department budgets.

A second argument relates to the cost of employing a volunteer organizer, as required for Stroke Association Dysphasic Support services. It might well be argued that additional speech and language therapy sessions would be a more appropriate use of limited resources. The distance of commissioners who make the main contracting decisions in the health care quasi-market from speech and language therapy (as noted in Chapter 6) may increase therapists' natural anxiety on this count about possible implications for the service they can offer.

The third argument is that the case for more speech and language therapy posts is weakened if their work is (at least apparently) reduced by the employment of volunteers (Foggitt, 1987). However, a counter argument against this last claim is the idea that where volunteers are involved 'in the main stroke awareness is raised and more patients are referred, needing more speech and language therapists' (E.J. Innes, 1995, personal communication).

Negative impact on the speech and language therapy profession

There is a danger that volunteer involvement may have the effect of downgrading speech and language therapy (Foggitt, 1987). To avoid potential deskilling of the profession, it is essential to be clear that volunteers do not have the expertise to provide speech and language therapy.

ROLES FOR VOLUNTEERS WITH APHASIC PEOPLE

As we have shown, many speech and language therapists do deploy volunteers with their aphasic patients, or refer people to another organization that manages volunteers. The rest of this chapter is therefore concerned with how volunteers are deployed and with ways to promote good practice.

To some extent, roles of volunteers working with individuals will differ from those in groups, but there are considerable overlaps. Most groups run to a regular pattern that includes: small group/individual work with a volunteer, refreshments, games, a quiz or other larger group activities and perhaps physical exercises. Many clubs go on outings from time to time, providing aphasic people with the opportunity to eat in a pub or restaurant, or visit a place of interest. Volunteers working with individuals may also have outings, sometimes a trip to the local shops or to a nearby town, or to pursue a shared interest. A volunteer may combine two or more roles in one activity and/or at different times. What, then, are these roles?

Communication practice

Communication practice is provided by volunteers with individuals and groups. A useful distinction can be made between **therapy practice** and **communication maintenance**, and we discuss each in turn.

Therapy practice is carried out under the direction of a speech and language therapist, in order to consolidate work done during therapy sessions. This was the most frequent volunteer activity reported in the CSLT Aphasia Working Party national survey, with 68% of districts using volunteers deploying at least some of them in this way (Mackenzie *et al.*, 1993). The therapist provides the volunteer with a specific programme of work to this end. An example of this was the co-operation of a Stroke Association Dysphasic Support volunteer with the speech and language therapist to help a young mother who, following a stroke, was receiving speech and language therapy twice a week. The speech and language therapist and volunteer shared an exercise book so that each could see the work the other was doing, and the therapist asked the volunteer to undertake specific tasks, week by week.

Therapy practice is usually conducted on a one-to-one basis, in the aphasic person's home or within a group. We have seen that speech and language therapists opposed to volunteers argue that it is more appropriate for relatives than for volunteers to provide therapy practice, an issue we discuss further in Chapter 9. Therapists who favour volunteers would argue that even where the family is providing communication practice, patients can benefit from the additional contact that volunteers offer.

Communication maintenance may take place alongside speech and language therapy or after an aphasic person has been discharged from speech and language therapy. The aim is to provide continuing practice in order to prevent the aphasic person's communication from deteriorating. Communication maintenance is often less closely supervised by a speech and language therapist than is therapy practice. With individuals, opportunities for communication may be afforded by the volunteer facilitating outings to wherever the aphasic person wants to go, be it to play dominoes, bingo, or bridge, or to visit a public house, social club or restaurant. Many therapists see groups as particularly appropriate for communication maintenance. Their value is in helping aphasic people to apply whatever language and other communication skills they possess in a relaxed, enjoyable social situation, thus improving their 'functional communication'.

Ancillary tasks

In group settings there are a number of ancillary tasks such as transport, refreshments, taking coats and helping people to their chairs, which volunteers can take on, thus freeing others to spend more time working on language.

Social contact

Volunteers can provide a social outlet for aphasic people. We have discussed the often damaging effects of aphasia on social relationships in Chapter 2. A volunteer's visits and/or weekly club meeting are events aphasic people can look forward to and enjoy, thus helping to maintain their morale and enhance their quality of life. A volunteer may contribute in providing social contact, whether or not there is any conscious focus on social skills. A spillover effect is also possible: The Stroke Association experience has been that, once their volunteers have set the example, friends and neighbours begin to visit. There may also be other benefits. Lesser and Watt's study (1978), mentioned at the beginning of this chapter, concluded that 'all the assessments confirmed ... an increase in social confidence' (p. 1047). From a service management perspective, referral to a voluntary scheme is a way of easing discharge from therapy for patients.

Continuing social support

Volunteers can go beyond this role to give continuing social support to aphasic people. Offering friendship can benefit an aphasic person in several ways. First, the volunteer is someone new who has chosen to take an interest, rather than being paid to provide treatment or care.

Second, the aphasic person's relationship with a volunteer is inherently different from that with carers. As one speech and language therapist explained:

> Communication handicaps can be very isolating, however skilled a communicator the handicapped person is. Communication with carers is often restricted to functional communication. A new person may be able to communicate at a more stimulating, more personally rewarding level. The new contact has different expectations about the handicapped person from carers. A person with a communication handicap is likely to have very few opportunities for meeting new people, limited opportunities to do ... things such as going swimming, going to an exhibition, or metal-detecting. This is partly due to the preconceptions of others, and partly due to other handicaps.

It may also be easier for aphasic people to accept their 'new selves' with volunteers, who cannot make comparisons with the past, but accept the people they are now.

Third, there are practical ways in which volunteers can help. Volunteers may accompany aphasic people to (for instance) dental appointments, to represent them, act as interpreters, and liaise with others who may find it difficult to communicate with them.

Communication maintenance on an individual basis, and the social outlet and support roles may be of particular importance for aphasic people in residential accommodation. One study in Australia concluded that:

> A ... benefit of using volunteers ... was the establishment of a social network outside the nursing home for the residents involved in the project. Volunteers have continued contact with group members on an informal basis since completing the programme, and both residents and volunteers have reported positive gains from a personal perspective as a result of these continuing relationships.

(Jordan et al., 1993, p. 80)

Support for relatives

So far, we have considered volunteers' roles in relation to people who have aphasia themselves. Volunteers can also provide support for relatives. Aphasic people's attendance at a club or centre for a day or even a couple of hours gives carers precious time to themselves to catch up with the shopping, go to the hairdressers, or pursue an interest that the aphasic person does not or cannot share. For many, this will be their only break from a mentally and physically exhausting and emotionally draining responsibility. The regular attendance of a home-visiting volunteer may serve a similar purpose: the partner does not feel guilty if she or he goes out while the volunteer is there, as the aphasic person is engaged in constructive activity rather than merely being left with a 'sitter'

Volunteers can provide support for relatives in more positive ways. Relatives may well be involved in club outings, and in some instances are invited into the club for part of the day and/or for special occasions. The Stroke Association has found that a spouse will often select one volunteer as confidant, and may contact this volunteer to talk over any problems that arise. Such a relationship is something that has to develop over time. Some Dysphasic Support services make more formal provision for supporting relatives. One arrangement is to hold a carer's group meeting concurrently with the Dysphasic Support group, in another room at the same venue, perhaps on a monthly or quarterly basis. This might simply be a social gathering or include a speaker from one of the caring professions. Another pattern is for evening meetings to be held for carers. Volunteers are also involved in The Stroke Association Community Services, Family Support, which is described in Chapter 9.

WHAT MAKES A GOOD VOLUNTEER?

Speech and language therapists, volunteer organizers, other volunteers and aphasic people all contribute to a volunteer's success.

Volunteers themselves will not necessarily have specific skills to offer, although some do. Many of the early VSS volunteers had been nurses or teachers (Griffith, 1975) but more recently one local organizer we spoke to suggested that teachers do not always make good volunteers, who need 'an informal, laid back attitude'. Another club organizer commented on helpers: 'Although several have come from the caring professions I find that the personality of the individual is *far* more important than formal training or past hospital experience.'

Characteristics looked for in volunteers suggest that approaches vary considerably. Griffith, writing about the early days of the CHSA VSS, stated that 'common sense, the ability to observe, and the desire to help were the only requirements' (1975). A speech and language therapist with responsibility for organizing a British Red Cross scheme looked for 'intuitive, kindly people who are humble and not patronising'. A speech and language therapist responsible for volunteer recruitment at a Communication Aid Centre suggested that: 'Volunteers need to be sensitive, intelligent, imaginative, reliable, and to have stamina, self-confidence, interest'. Other qualities mentioned to us were: insight, the ability to empathize, tolerance and flexibility.

These differing views each have important implications in relation to the recruitment and selection of volunteers. Most speech and language therapists we spoke to emphasized that it was essential to be selective. This view is strongly reinforced by the CSLT (1991) in their statement that: 'the selection procedure should be no less rigorous' than that for paid speech and language therapy assistants (p.279). This may be difficult to ensure where volunteers are recruited by voluntary organizations, which may be reluctant to turn down offers of help. Selection does take place, to a certain extent, within the more comprehensive schemes as volunteers are steered towards the most appropriate task for them, whether it be work with aphasic people at a club, tea making, driving, home visits to work on language, social visits or fundraising.

Recruitment and selection methods vary from the informal asking of friends and acquaintances to advertisements in the local or national press, on local radio or in a community centre. One speech and language therapist sometimes recruited volunteers for particular clients, and would then specify in some detail the kind of person required. She did ask for references, something individual Stroke Association Dysphasic Support services are increasingly doing. The roles of volunteer bureaux vary. Some take responsibility for obtaining references and conducting initial interviews to determine the kind of work for which a volunteer is best suited; others simply advertise vacancies. Those recruiting volunteers interviewed potential recruits, enabling the volunteer to learn more about what was required as well as allowing assessment of the volunteer's suitability. The most stringent selection process we encountered was at a speech and language club that required references and an interview first at the local volunteer bureau and then at the club. Volunteers were taken on initially for a 6-week trial period, after which those accepted signed a simple contract.

A good volunteer will be someone who thoroughly enjoys the work and the people, and has a genuine interest in learning from aphasic people about their lives, experiences and interests. Those organizing volunteers stress the commitment necessary, and those fearful of involving volunteers see this as a problem. However, the actual experience everywhere was that volunteers were prepared to make a regular commitment and honour it, with many choosing to exceed this commitment. The work made volunteers feel useful and needed, and put aspects of their own lives into perspective. One volunteer wrote about the club where she worked:

> Twelve o'clock comes round, all too soon. Some may think that I have given my time but am I really the giver or the RECEIVER ...? I go home, fully inspired and the housework that seemed a mountain earlier on, now seems a molehill.
>
> *(Camp n.d., p. 10)*

Volunteers' attitudes towards people with aphasia are extremely important. The volunteer must respect aphasic people and see them as equals. Patronizing or condescending attitudes have negative effects. Disabled people too need to feel needed, to help each other. Volunteers anxious to minister to their every need deny them the opportunity to use their own initiative to help themselves or other people.

Volunteers also need to appreciate the limitations of their role. It is inappropriate for volunteers to give advice to relatives about communication, or to comment to them on the overall progress of the aphasic person, for example, since these tasks require the speech and language therapist's expertise. If volunteers make such comments, they are likely to give a glowing report. The speech and language therapist has to provide a realistic assessment that may well be less favourable, and which relatives may therefore be less inclined to accept. The volunteer can thus undermine the speech and language therapist's position in relation to an aphasic person's family.

The volunteer will probably spend more time with the aphasic person than the speech and language therapist can afford. The setting for this contact is likely to be a relaxed one, either the aphasic person's own home or a friendly club. The speech and language therapist may see the patient in a clinical setting, or even if there is a home visit the patient and carer may be reluctant to 'waste' precious therapy time by raising problems that they see as not being directly related to communication. Some patients and/or families, then, will give a volunteer a far better picture of the problems they are experiencing than is available to the therapist. Should the volunteer pass such information on to the therapist? The volunteer may feel that to do so will constitute a breach of trust, but on the other hand the information may help the therapist to treat the patient more effectively. It is clearly a matter of judgment for the volunteer. The best approach is for the volunteer to be as open as possible with the aphasic person and family, so that information is channelled to the speech and language therapist with their full knowledge and approval and becomes, in effect, an extra link between them.

This issue of confidentiality occurs also in the opposite direction. Speech and language therapists may give information to volunteers that is solely for their use, rather than to be passed on. These situations raise the important issue of the precise nature of the three or four-way relationship between the aphasic person, volunteer, speech and language therapist and, possibly, carer/ relatives. Stroke Association volunteers sign a statement on confidentiality.

In order to work confidently, volunteers need to understand both their own role and that of the therapist. To a considerable extent it must be the speech and language therapist's responsibility to define expectations, and to communicate these to volunteers, preferably both verbally and in writing. The Bury Speakeasy Club *Volunteers' Handbook* (1988b) shows that it is possible for even local schemes to specify expectations in a friendly, non-threatening way. Where another organization is involved the volunteer organizer also has a part to play here. One such organizer describes her approach:

> I often tell my volunteers that we work best when using our own common sense and kindliness. Empathy and compassion for others help us enormously. It is very important that we do not lose our essential neighbourly ease of manner. We do not patronise, we do not diagnose, we do not make easy promises. We do not pretend to be doctors, counsellors nor speech and language therapists. In this sense we are all amateurs – but not amateurish.
>
> (*Leroy, 1992, p. 8*)

Particularly in relation to those people continuing with therapy, close coordination between the therapist and the volunteer is essential, whether or not the volunteer works directly for the speech and language therapy department. More generally, good back-up support for volunteers and organizers is important both to ensure that the service provided is of the highest possible quality and to retain volunteers' interest. Volunteers need both organizational and peer group support. Organizational support can best be provided by scheme organizers and by having an identified speech and language therapist who takes responsibility for liaising with each scheme. This role might involve, as in one local scheme visited, assessment of all new referrals to the clubs, visiting each club about once a month and keeping in contact with the organizers in order to deal with any day-to-day problems that may arise. Some clubs set aside a time for volunteers to talk to each other away from members. Training sessions and social occasions may also afford opportunities for peer group support.

Supervision of volunteers presents fewer problems in a group or club than in relation to home visiting. The Stroke Association Dysphasic Support local organizers have regular progress meetings for the home-visiting volunteers who see each patient, to which they invite the speech and language therapist. Organizers are advised to contact a volunteer after the first home visit to ask how things went and to make sure there are no problems, and volunteers can contact the organizer by phone to discuss any difficulties that may arise later.

Those people managing volunteers need to offer support and advice, but it is up to the volunteers themselves to accept this. It is important that volunteers respect the speech and language therapist's expertise and recognize how little they themselves know about the technical aspects of helping people with aphasia. Good volunteers are willing to learn and take any opportunity to do so. They know when they are out of their depth and realize that they will make mistakes. They therefore seek advice. There is a danger that as volunteers gain experience and become familiar with a few speech and language therapy concepts they overreach themselves, assuming that they 'know it all'. One example came from a speech and language therapist who asks volunteers to observe a patient's therapy before becoming one of that person's home visitors. In one instance an experienced volunteer did not do so. Her first home visit was a disaster: she kept the work too simple, and so upset the aphasic person that the arrangement had to be abandoned. Pitching sessions either too low or too high can be very frustrating for aphasic people, and can undermine their confidence. Some volunteers use tasks, games, etc. which aphasic adults will define as childish and which damage their self-esteem, while the volunteer appears as patronizing. Another common area of difficulty relates to comprehension problems. Many aphasic people whose comprehension is incomplete are skilled at masking this, perhaps by giving non-verbal indications that they do follow what is being said. Volunteers sometimes wrongly insist that the aphasic person can understand everything.

Liaison between a speech and language therapist, if possible one with responsibility for adult services, and the local organizer is the main link between Stroke Association Dysphasic Support and speech and language therapy departments. The Stroke Association local organizers we met valued highly the speech and language therapist's advice, and our impression is that Dysphasic Support as a whole is moving towards closer co-operation with the speech and language therapy profession, something that is to be welcomed. The local organizer must give a lead to the volunteers in developing a close relationship with speech and language therapists if the kinds of problems outlined above are to be avoided.

TRAINING FOR VOLUNTEERS

Practice as regards training of volunteers varies widely (Jordan, 1989b), sometimes even within schemes. The training provided for Stroke Association volunteers, for example, varies partly according to the support and availability of speech and language therapists and how much time they can give. The Stroke Association uses its own contacts and staff to provide training if speech and language therapists are not available. In one of the two (then) VSSs we visited, the speech and language therapy department took responsibility for this training. In the other, training sessions were provided, for home-visiting volunteers only, by the local organizer. We now consider, in turn, approaches to training and its organization and the aims and content of training.

Approaches to training and its organization

We distinguish between four models:

- No training: Of therapists responding to the survey of Mackenzie *et al.* (1993) 21% of those using assistants or volunteers 'stated that no training was provided' (p. 47). One reason for volunteers not receiving any training is that it is seen as unnecessary. This appears to have been the view of the VSS in the past. Its volunteers would 'go into the homes [of patients] as friendly neighbours' (Griffith and Miller, 1980). Briefings and follow-up meetings with the local organizer and other volunteers visiting a given patient were (and are) arranged. More generally, evidence we collected suggests that where training is seen as desirable, it is not always provided, perhaps owing to 'lack of time'. In some instances, training sessions at the start of a scheme were not repeated for absentees or for later joiners, who might be expected to 'learn the ropes' by assisting an experienced volunteer.
- Informal training: Particularly in rural areas, there may be too few volunteers to create a viable training group. In one area the new volunteer was treated like a student, observing therapy sessions (with the patient's agreement) and discussing each session with the therapist afterwards. Informal training may be most appropriate in equipping the volunteer for work with a particular client.
- Workshop approach: This might involve a single training session, occasional training days, or an ongoing series. One example encountered was a half-day session provided by a speech and language therapist for six to eight new volunteers to a (then) VSS. Another involved several speech clubs in a predominantly rural area joining forces for occasional training days. A third was an annual programme of two county-wide training days and four more local sessions for volunteers to an ABE service run by the local authority education department in one county. ABE volunteers might also work in groups to produce materials packs. Three speech and language therapy services in the county of Devon have agreed a common training protocol for Dysphasic Support service volunteers. This involves a half-day training session for all new volunteers run by a senior speech and language therapist, annual large group sessions (again run by a therapist) and review sessions in which volunteers share information with the speech and language therapist who knows the clients in order to help evaluate progress, learn from the therapist and plan for the future (Spencer, 1994).

- Training courses: One advantage of a large scheme is in recruiting enough new volunteers to justify fairly frequent training courses. In one club with a total of about 40 volunteers, new volunteers spend a probationary period of 6 weeks in the club, observing members and joining in group activities, before attending a 2-day basic training course. In addition, all volunteers are invited to attend refresher training sessions held each year. The club's *Volunteer Handbook* states clearly that: 'Volunteers are expected to attend training and support sessions. This is for everybody's benefit' (Speakeasy Club, 1994b, p. 6).

Educational institutions are a potential source of volunteer training courses on working with aphasic people. Apart from education-based schemes providing training for their own volunteers, this source has, to date, been little explored in Britain. An exception has been the Department of Clinical Communication Studies at London's City University. It offered three short courses during the later half of the 1980s and a further course in 1992. Each catered for some ten to 15 students, giving a total of around 50 students completing one of these four courses. Volunteers were 'referred' through ADA, from the (then) VSS and by speech and language therapists. They thus came from a range of different organizations and schemes. City University's central position gave the courses a wide catchment area, spanning greater London and the home counties. The format of the course varied; for example, the last of the three intakes in the 1980s (1988) attended nine 2-hour weekly sessions, whilst the 1992 course was for 1 week. This latter course was run in collaboration with ADA.

Aims and content of training

The Speakeasy Club (1994b) describes the twofold aim of its volunteer training as follows:

> Obviously, it is important [for volunteers] to have some background knowledge of language disorder and how it affects the member; but also, we feel it is very important for Speakeasy volunteers to have some training in communication skills ... The aim of this is to provide a climate in which people with speech problems can feel valued and function effectively.
>
> *(p. 5)*

Speakeasy's basic training course uses a range of teaching methods: videos, talks and discussions, ideally with some input from an aphasic person. Content includes: discussion of the nature of speech and language disorders and how best to help communication-impaired people to communicate; an introduction to alternative means of communication; the role of speech and language therapists; a session on developing listening skills; guidance on adapting topic-based projects and worksheets to the needs of different aphasic people; and advice on how to handle a wheelchair. Past City University courses covered broadly similar areas. In addition, their location in the department running the City Dysphasic Group enabled practical experience to be built into the course. Participants were able to observe a speech and language therapist running a group and then to do so themselves, receiving feedback on this. Video clips of aphasic people talking were also used as a basis for structured tasks such as identification of different communication strategies. Whilst training for Stroke Association Dysphasic Support volunteers is, as indicated above, determined in each locality, its centrally provided guidelines cover similar ground to the Speakeasy training.

At City University, ideas have changed somewhat as to the most appropriate aims and content for future courses. They will focus more on the need to empower aphasic people. Volunteers will be encouraged to examine prevalent attitudes towards disability and their own attitudes both towards aphasic people and in relation to volunteering. The objectives will be to increase awareness of potentially patronizing attitudes and forms of behaviour, and of participants' motivations for volunteering and what they gain from being a volunteer. The plan is to engage aphasic people as trainers of volunteers. Follow-up, monitoring and training of volunteers on the job are also considered necessary to reinforce changes in volunteers' attitudes and approach. (C. Pound, 1995, personal communication) Such follow-up might well prove difficult if participants come from a number of different volunteer schemes and from different areas.

In general, our findings suggest that:

- speech and language therapists are concerned about volunteer training and accept a responsibility in this;
- many volunteers welcome the opportunity to learn more about the work;
- a range of formats is being used in different situations, giving very varied amounts of training;
- there has so far been much common ground as regards content (Jordan, 1989b);
- ideas derived from the social model of disability are beginning to influence thinking about the form and content of volunteer training, but may have yet to be put into practice in Britain.

GOOD PRACTICE GUIDELINES

The extent and nature of volunteer involvement with aphasic people varies considerably from area to area in Britain (Jordan, 1989a, 1991). The CSLT (1991) comments that 'numerous services would be non operational were it not for the support of their volunteers; (p. 279). Speech and language therapy departments have brought in volunteers partly because they believe they can contribute towards meeting aphasic people's needs, and partly to ease their own shortfalls of resources in relation to those needs. The balance between the 'needs' and 'resources' elements will have affected the decision as to whether or not to involve volunteers at all and the way any volunteer scheme operates. It may be significant that it was in the two understaffed districts of the three studied by Jordan (1991) that speech and language therapists had volunteers working with them, whilst one of the main reasons for not involving volunteers in therapy put forward by speech and language therapists in the better-staffed district was that they would not have time to train them properly!

It should be a matter of professional concern if the resource argument is dominant, both because of the costs necessary if a volunteer scheme is to be satisfactory, and because it is in this situation that aphasia therapy itself can most easily be undermined. To bring in volunteers, or a volunteer scheme, in such circumstances may be an abnegation of speech therapists' responsibility to treat aphasic people.

The purchaser/provider split, with its underlying philosophy of competition among providers for contracts as a means of achieving maximal cost-effectiveness, raises the possibility of volunteer organizations approaching purchasers in direct competition to statutory services. Decisions regarding the introduction of volunteer schemes would then be made by purchasers far removed from any particular service and, in theory, such decisions could be taken without reference to speech and language therapy managers. Services involving volunteers have an inbuilt cost advantage, as well as promoting 'skill mix' – a fashionable concept in recent years. In practice, such a situation is unlikely to occur, given the stated intention of the largest organization in this field to open a service only with the approval of the local speech and language therapy management. A more probable scenario is of statutory and voluntary providers working together to present a proposal that incorporates both service elements to the health commissioning body. As explained in Chapter 6, one of the inevitable effects of the changes in NHS management is that policies and procedures will differ even more than before from one area to another. We lack anything approaching a complete picture, both generally (see Chapter 5) and in relation to volunteer deployment with aphasic people.

Contracts can act as a quality assurance tool at local level, and it is highly desirable that such matters as recruitment procedures for volunteers and measures to maintain confidentiality should be specified in them. Clear guidance to speech and language therapists working with volunteer schemes can provide further protection for aphasic people. Spencer (1994) has developed practical guidelines for therapists working with Stroke Association volunteers in the South Devon Healthcare Trust. These cover: referrals, introducing patients to volunteers, volunteer training, monitoring, contact with the scheme organizer, written reports, discharge from the scheme and the role of the volunteer. In general, quality control guidelines are needed:

- to cover the process of volunteering (this includes recruitment, selection, supervision, monitoring and training);
- to set parameters for volunteers' roles and 'conditions of service' (Jordan, 1990).

Such guidelines would need to identify the ideal, existing best practice and acceptable minima. They would cover, for example, whether references should be required for all volunteers or only for home-visiting volunteers.

Some of the issues have already been the subject of professional consideration at national level. The CST Aphasia Working Party (1989) stated that 'volunteers ... should ... complement rather than supplement the speech therapy service to aphasic people' and calls for speech therapy managers to develop a clear policy regarding volunteers (p. 7). More recently the CSLT's professional standards document, *Communicating Quality* (1991) advised speech and language therapy services ' ... to work in close conjunction with volunteer schemes which may be in operation' and called for 'training opportunities available to the volunteers [to] reflect the expectations of their role' (p. 279). ADA holds the view that any involvement of volunteers in language work with patients should be under the direct supervision of a speech and language therapist and that all volunteers should receive training.

The aim must be to ensure that volunteer projects or schemes achieve a satisfactory outcome for all parties involved: aphasic people, carers, volunteers, volunteer organizers and professionals. Speech and language therapists should look to the RCSLT to develop national guidelines. This could be done most productively in consultation with the main voluntary organizations concerned.

VOLUNTEERING BASED ON THE SOCIAL MODEL OF DISABILITY: THE APHASIA CENTRE – NORTH YORK, CANADA

In Chapter 4 we outlined the theoretical underpinnings of the Aphasia Centre – North York approach and located the Centre's work in the social model of disability. We described the Centre's concern with removing the social barriers that limit aphasic people's access to everyday conversation. Here we focus on volunteer involvement.

The North York Centre began in 1979 as a volunteer organization – a group of three volunteers and seven aphasic people. It was a response by Pat Arato to the lack of long-term community speech and language therapy available to her husband, who had become aphasic following a stroke in

1978. Pat Arato's inspiration came from a lecture by Valerie Eaton Griffith and the actress Patricia Neal, whose experience led to the setting up of what is now known as the Stroke Association Dysphasic Support service in Britain and to similar services elsewhere, as described at the beginning of this chapter. The presentation focused on 'the potential for using volunteers to provide support for people with aphasia' (Kagan and Gailey, 1993, p. 201). By 1994 the Centre had grown to 200 members and 130 volunteers. (Aphasia Centre – North York, 1994a) It has a staff of ten (5 full-time and 5 part-time) including a volunteer coordinator and several speech–language pathologists. Speech–language pathologists have been employed at the Centre since 1984 (ibid.). The Centre is financed partly by the provincial government and in part from its own fundraising. Its service is different from and complementary to speech–language pathology. The Centre provides communication opportunities and continuing community support for as long as aphasic members wish to or are able to attend. Members usually attend 2 days a week. Since the late 1980s there have been two satellite centres in different parts of Ontario, one in the rural area of Stouffville and the other in Ottawa.

Most of the North York Centre's volunteers are women drawn from very wide age, educational and vocational bands. Volunteers undergo rigorous training and most then attend 1 day a week (Kagan and Gailey, 1993). Opportunities for volunteers at the Centre include working directly with aphasic members or providing support services. The latter comprise receptionist and office work, staffing the gift shop, fundraising, organizing special events such as awareness campaigns and committee work (Kagan and Gailey, 1993; Aphasia Centre – North York, 1994b). We concentrate here on volunteers' work directly with members.

The Centre's core communication programme runs on four mornings a week. Volunteers act as communication facilitators within small conversation groups of three to five aphasic members. In order to carry out this role, volunteers have to learn techniques:

- to facilitate aphasic members' understanding;
- to help them get their message across to the volunteer or another aphasic member;
- to maintain the feel and flow of conversation (Kagan and Gailey, 1993).

Resources on each group's table include, for example, photographs of group members and staff, number and alphabet boards, a colour chart, maps, paper and pencils, and daily papers. There is a theme for each session and theme-related pictographs and key words are also provided (ibid.). Recreational activities such as painting, crafts, cards, singing, and exercise are provided in afternoon sessions. These are regarded as providing further opportunities for conversation, and the volunteers assisting in these sessions are also trained communication facilitators.

Most of the North York speech–language pathologists' time is spent in training volunteers (Arato and Kagan, 1995). Newly recruited volunteers do at least 12 hours' observation over 5 weeks, and undergo 17 intensive hours of training. They then begin to work with groups under close supervision. Formal training ends only when the speech–language pathologist and the volunteer both evaluate the latter's level of skills as satisfactory (ibid; Kagan and Gailey, 1993).The training includes discussion of such issues as:

- the distinction between 'practicing techniques to facilitate conversation', the aim of which is to improve functional communication skills, and 'providing conversational opportunity' whose goal is improved psychosocial well-being;
- awareness of group members' severity levels and their varied abilities to use compensatory techniques;
- the need to avoid slipping into a teaching role, rather than that of facilitator;
- how to talk for aphasic members, orchestrating conversation and helping to convey members' messages, rather than taking over (Kagan and Gailey, 1993, pp. 216–17).

The complexity and difficulty of some of the concepts and techniques introduced for volunteers are recognized, as is the need for continuous support, monitoring, supervision and reinforcement of the Centre's philosophy (ibid.). Special training is required to enable volunteers to work with aphasic people who have severe difficulties in understanding accompanied by fluent speech (p. 211). Volunteers meet with speech–language pathologists at the beginning and end of each morning, for briefing and reporting back respectively. The speech–language pathologists move among the groups during the morning, and are available to discuss any problems with the volunteers during the mid-morning break.

The achievement of the North York Aphasia Centre is described by an English visitor. In relation to volunteers: 'An atmosphere is engendered in which the contribution the volunteers can make to the development of the materials and tasks is taken seriously and a real sharing of ideas and concerns takes place' (Byng, 1990, p. 14), whilst as regards aphasic people's position: 'The whole emphasis of the group is changed from traditionally placing the onus on the aphasics to modify their communication to requiring those around the aphasic person to know how to facilitate the communication skills that the aphasic person has available' . The volunteers take on the important role of 'communication ramps' (Kagan and Gailey, 1993, p. 204), enabling aphasic people to participate in, share responsibility for and enjoy conversation. As discussed in Chapter 4, Kagan's analysis (1995) emphasizes the centrality of conversation for self-esteem and hence psychosocial well-being.

Endnotes

[1]As explained in Chapter 5, in England and Wales there have been name changes of both the charity and this particular service, which has become the 'Stroke Association Community Services, Dysphasic Support'.

[2]Schemes recruiting volunteers vary in their selection criteria. People with some of the conditions described here are not eligible as volunteers for all schemes.

PART THREE

People, Policies and Power

Social model aphasia therapy | 8

Aphasia therapy, as we have shown, is founded almost exclusively in an individual pathology model of disability. We have also demonstrated, however, mainly by describing developments at the Aphasia Centre – North York in Canada, that it is possible to orientate intervention to the removal of social barriers. In this chapter we explore the case for change and the implications of adopting a social model mind set. We are concerned with both what is needed and how it can best be achieved. We start by considering the arguments against individual pathology-based professional practice. We then review the individual and social models of disability as they apply to aphasia therapy, and focus on professional practice, the issue of resources, the working environment of speech and language therapists and research.

CRITIQUES OF PROFESSIONAL PRACTICE

The literature considering services from disabled people's perspectives includes little reference to speech and language therapy, and none to aphasia. This is not surprising given, for example, the small size of the profession and the barriers aphasic people have to overcome to contribute in this arena. Discussions of health and welfare professionals in general show that, at worst, professional practice can be experienced by disabled people as 'dehumanising and abusive' (French, 1994b, p. 103). Professionals are in a position to wield a considerable amount of power over disabled people, for example by defining their needs, determining their access to resources, 'managing' interactions with them and controlling many aspects of their lives (ibid. pp. 103, 109; Oliver, 1990). Barnes (1991) calls rehabilitation services 'highly discriminatory and a disservice to disabled people' (p. 131) and states that rehabilitation is 'not only a product of institutional discrimination against disabled people; it is also a central component in the discriminatory process' (ibid.). This is because rehabilitative services aim to help disabled people function in the face of economic, environmental and social barriers that remedial therapists accept as given and because the rehabilitation process places disabled people in a role of dependency (ibid., p. 132), giving them no opportunity to contribute towards policy or practice (French, 1994b). Finkelstein (1991) sheds some light on the process by which professions have come to earn the disability movement's indictment, showing that professionals' position is an unintended consequence of (misguided) attempts to help disabled people:

> The administrative 'cure and care' approach to disability set service providers apart from those who they wished to serve under the illusion that they were being 'objective'. We now see this 'professionalism' as having legitimised the imposition of able-bodied assumptions that to have a disability is to experience a form of social death. In this respect the promoters and defenders of existing services can themselves often be experienced as disabling barriers inhibiting the control of disabled people over their own lives.'
>
> *(p. 35)*

Aphasia therapists' position and status certainly mean that they might act in the ways described above. The CSLT professional guidelines (1991), however, promote a partnership approach which should strongly discourage excessive use of professional power. Aphasia therapy located firmly in the individual pathology model of disability may lack sensitivity to social barriers that limit communication. It is possible that at least some such therapy nevertheless does provide services that have the effect of reducing some barriers, for example through advice to family members about communication strategies to employ. Understanding of the social model provides a new theoretical justification for such work and, as we have indicated (pp. 60–2 and 130–2), calls for an extension in therapist's responsibilities.

French (1994b) and Oliver (1990) point out that professionals are by no means free agents, being 'as much trapped in dependency-creating relationships as are their [disabled] clients' (Oliver, 1990, p. 91) and that professionals are the more dependent, relying on disabled people for their livelihood (ibid.). Policies to institute equal rights for disabled people are needed at different levels within organizations. The Living Options Partnership (funded jointly by the King's Fund Centre and the Prince of Wales Advisory Group on Disability) discussed issues and good practice concerning disabled people's involvement in the health commissioning process (Morris, 1995) and produced a guide for senior managers (Begum and Fletcher, 1995). Even without such policies, however, individual professionals can practise in ways to empower service users (French, 1994b).

MODELS OF DISABILITY AND APHASIA THERAPY REVISITED

As we saw in Chapter 4, aphasia therapy fits easily into the individual pathology-based WHO typology of impairment, disability and handicap. Impairment level therapy is concerned with the component parts of language, whilst therapy at disability level means assisting aphasic people to communicate in the real world. Handicap level therapy involves emotional support, and also indirect help by enabling an aphasic person's significant others to improve their ability to communicate with that aphasic person. This may be taken a step further as, for example, at the North York Aphasia Centre where health professionals and volunteers undertake a training programme to facilitate their communication with aphasic people more generally. Kagan (1995) describes their approach in terms of the WHO classification and sees her work as addressing the handicap of aphasia.

The social model of disability places its main emphasis on factors in the environment that prevent disabled people's full participation in society. Its twofold categorization leads to the concept of impairment being heavily loaded, as it has to encompass both the damage to the body and the functional effects of this damage. Disability is defined entirely in terms of barriers, which may be physical, economic, social or psychological. Removing such barriers is seen as an essential prerequisite for the empowerment of aphasic people. Since communication means interpersonal interaction, it follows that a fruitful approach to overcoming the barriers that constitute, according to the social model, the disability of aphasia lies in enabling non-aphasic people to act as communication ramps. What are the implications of this model for aphasia therapy?

DISABILITY LEVEL PRACTICE THE SOCIAL MODEL WAY

The social model calls for an extension of aphasia services into using speech and language therapy expertise to train as wide a range of people as possible to communicate with aphasic people. This is, in the main, a new task for aphasia therapists. A first step is to raise awareness of aphasia and provide training among colleagues in health and social services. In Britain, such work was pioneered by the 'Words Fail Me' project in Sheffield. This was 'a training initiative for health authority staff ... aimed at improving the effectiveness of their communication with patients and colleagues' (Syder, 1989, p. 106). The project was concerned with four areas:

- the raising of professional awareness of the need for good communication generally;
- the presentation of simple strategies to enable staff to improve their own communication;
- the recognition and awareness of specific communication disorders in patients;
- improving interactions between patients with communication handicaps and members of staff.

(p. 107)

The project thus set the particular requirements for successful interactions with communication-impaired people alongside the more general need for good communication among staff and between staff and clientele in large, complex organizations. Outputs included:

- 'workshops on communication skills for any staff with patient contact', covering 'general communication skills and communication disorders'. The workshops were full day, small group, 'largely multi-unit and multi-disciplinary'. Over 900 people participated in them, including clinicians and others such as medical records staff;
- 'an information pack ... for clinical staff about adult communication disorders ... [This] has also been sold outside the district';
- a test to screen for aphasia for use by hospital doctors and GPs. The intention was to increase doctors' understanding of aphasia and so prevent non-diagnosis – and hence non-referral for treatment – in hospital and community.
- 'a symbol scheme ... for patients with communication disorders'. A logo was specially designed for display in health authority units whose staff had received training and patients were given a card to use;
- 'an extended communication skills course' for senior managerial staff.

(Syder, 1989, p. 107; Syder et al., 1993)

Whilst the 'Words Fail Me' project did not survive the departure of its initiator, some specific aspects have lasted in Sheffield and have been further advanced. The principle that training on communication disability should locate it in the framework of communication needs more generally is being applied in various contexts. Training is offered to residential care homes (Lester, Soord and Trewhitt, 1994), private nursing homes and day care centres. Some courses in Sheffield are provided for staff and service users together (Mangan and Trewhitt, 1993), and training on equal access to communication has also been developed (Trewhitt, 1995). The Sheffield programme has been a major influence on an ADA project aiming to produce and disseminate a training package on communication for formal and informal carers (pp. 172, 182).

Care staff may need initial support to enable them to develop specific services to foster communication. Bryan and Drew (1987) found that considerable speech and language therapist input was necessary to set up and manage communication groups in residential homes. A therapist worked alongside care staff for the first 6 weeks, after which the groups continued, with the speech and language therapist withdrawing to a monitoring role.

At the end of Chapter 7 we described the Aphasia Centre – North York approach to volunteer involvement and, in particular, the training of volunteers to become conversation partners for aphasic people. It might be argued that this in effect already happens in countless schemes involving volunteers in Britain. To some extent this may be so. Kagan's unique contribution is her development of a theoretical justification for speech and language therapists' training of volunteers (among others) to use specific strategies aimed at revealing aphasic people's masked competence. This gives a much sharper focus than hitherto. It confers on volunteers a more precisely defined role that is different from and complementary to that of the speech and language therapist. In Chapter 7 we set out the case against using volunteers. Most of the arguments presented there concerned the respective roles of therapists and volunteers, and thus fall away once these roles are clearly distinguished. One possible objection that remains pertains to a posited risk in exposing aphasic people to volunteers, for example through breaches in confidentiality. As we saw, this potential problem can largely be overcome by a combination of clear rules for volunteers, perhaps including a simple volunteer contract, and openness with aphasic people about the exchange of relevant personal and clinical information. Another aspect was concern about therapists' lack of control over volunteers. The North York Aphasia Centre is organized so as to provide volunteers with both supervision and support from speech and language therapists. Arato and Kagan (1995) emphasize the necessity of close monitoring as well as initial and ongoing training in order to maintain consistently the conversation partner role. Improving these aspects of volunteer schemes should be a major priority for speech and language therapists working with them.

The main objection to volunteer involvement on ethical grounds suggests that therapists should look instead to family members to assist aphasic people's language recovery (see pp. 116–17). As argued elsewhere (Jordan, 1989a) this oversimplifies the issue in several ways. For those aphasic people who live alone and are without nearby relatives, Foggitt (1987) suggests no alternative source of help. The ability of relatives to play a constructive part in language rehabilitation may be limited by a wide range of factors. For instance, power structures or attitudes toward disability within the family may not be conducive. In some close, long-standing relationships mutual understanding may reduce the need for words. Relationships – and relatives – under stress are also unlikely to pro-duce a favourable climate for 'therapy practice'. At the Aphasia Centre – North York, friends and relatives are advised not to attempt to take on a quasi-therapeutic role, but rather to learn the special communication skills required and then to get on with rebuilding a positive relationship with the aphasic person (1994b).

The relationship of volunteers to the aphasic people with whom they have contact differs in an important respect from those of both family and professionals. Family and friends have obligations towards aphasic people by virtue of pre-existing relationships, and professionals are paid to care. Volunteers' relationships with aphasic people are under no such constraints. They have chosen to make and maintain contact. This in itself may be singularly important to an aphasic person. Lyon (1989) refers to 'the apha-sic adults' perception that they are viable company with others who are not bound or committed to them' (p. 14).

Lyon's small study warrants further examination. His aim in enlisting volunteers to spend 4 to 6 hours a week with an aphasic person was 'to build a resource, a bridge, that might ultimately be used to activate or rekindle communicative desire ... for reasons outside the clinical setting' (p. 13). After about a month of meetings in the clinic, during which time each partner learnt specific communication strategies, the communication partners began to go out into the community to undertake activities chosen by the aphasic person. He reported on the first two pairings that all four participants had gained from the experience. The communica-tion partners' foremost gain was 'the realization that aphasic adults are, after all, only "ordinary people"' (p. 14). There are several instructive points to be made from Lyon's account. First, his underlying philosophy is, notwithstanding its different imagery, a social model one. Second, we should note what appears to be quite a considerable investment of speech and language therapy time. Finally, the volunteers' experience was educative for them; they learnt to see the person rather than the dis-ability.

IMPAIRMENT LEVEL PRACTICE UNDER THE SOCIAL MODEL

Despite their criticisms of health professionals' practice, disabled people accept that rehabilitation services directed at disabled people themselves can in some circumstances be appropriate. Major changes are called for, however. Finkelstein (1991) suggests that:

> the medical model and its rehabilitation service approach should always be determined in the context of the social (barriers) model and not vice versa ... This means that the extent, duration and nature of medical interventions should be guided by an understanding and analysis of the barriers to be overcome, rather than on the functional limitations of the individual.
>
> *(pp. 35–6)*

French (1994b) is even more direct, arguing that: 'To be truly effective health ... professionals must relinquish their power and control and work closely with disabled people under their direction (p. 111). The new role required is described as follows: 'workers in rehabilitation services should see themselves as a resource, to be tapped by disabled clients, rather than as professionals trained to make highly specialised assessments of what is appropriate for individual disabled people' (Finkelstein, 1991, p. 36). Working in a social model role, professionals 'do not attempt to dominate, to take control or to *manage* disabled people, but rather to act as supportive enablers, actively sharing their expertise and knowledge while recognizing the expertise of disabled people and learning from them' (French, 1994b, p. 115). Some skills more usually associated with counselling, in particular listening and feedback skills, will be valuable here. The professional's role also includes describing and illustrating to people the things that they are already doing that are facilitative, and supporting them in this, thus helping to reinforce empowering ways.

What kinds of service, then, do disabled people feel they need? A study of disabled people's needs and priorities in North Derbyshire concluded that 'disabled people wanted community services; they wanted information and more broadly based services, in areas such as peer counselling, rather than specific professional interventions' (Silburn, 1994, p. 251).

Aphasic people's and carers' felt need for information is illustrated in the final section of Chapter 6. The findings from Anderson's empirical study (1992) suggest that whilst professionals concerned with stroke patients are well aware that patients and carers require information and that sometimes their needs in this respect differ, 'probably fewer ... realise how these needs for information change over time'. He continues: 'This awareness was not translated into a systematic effort to inform. In particular, a majority of carers felt they had been ill-prepared for the events and experiences that followed the stroke' (pp. 223–4). Anderson acknowledges the difficulties professionals face in providing information given the variability of individual needs and preferences and uncertainty about the future but argues that, nevertheless:

> advice, information, support and encouragement should be at the centre of strategies to enhance the quality of life of patients and their carers. The focus of services cannot be upon the repair of underlying physical damage or even remedial therapy; it needs to be committed on a continuing basis to improving education and training for living with chronic illness. This implies better education and training for service providers: so that nurses, for example, can become more sensitive to the needs and experience of patients; so that staff can listen and talk together with the patients and their carers, identifying preferences for information (acknowledging that some patients, especially those who are older and more disabled, may not wish to cope with too much information) and preferences for caring. There is a need for service providers to recognise differences between their perceptions and those of others if they are to bridge the existing gaps in communication.
>
> *(p. 224)*

In relation to aphasia, the first need is for information about the disorder. Speech and language therapy expertise is essential here, given the complexity of aphasia, and explanations need to be backed up by written material. Some speech and language therapy departments produce their own leaflets but many distribute those produced by specialists within voluntary organizations (see Appendix B). There is also a need for full information about any intervention. In Chapter 5 we discussed the issue of negotiated treatment contracts, and the exchange of information they involve. All information must be provided in a form that aphasic people and their families find accessible and acceptable in order for any shift of power to service users to take place.

Silburn's findings in North Derbyshire suggest that disabled people's felt need for **counselling** might best be met by other disabled people, and we have described the beginnings in Britain of counselling of aphasic people by aphasic people in Chapter 4. We saw in Chapter 5 that some speech and language therapists also act as counsellors. Counselling may be justifiable as part of speech and language therapy to enable the aphasic person to benefit from treatment. Otherwise, referral to other agencies is likely to be more appropriate.

The North Derbyshire results call into question whether aphasic people want 'conventional' speech and language therapy directed at modifying their use of language and helping them to develop alternative means of communication. Some people do refuse aphasia therapy, but there is plenty of evidence of demand. A study of the experience of 28 people recently discharged from a hospital stroke unit in Kent of 'becoming consumers of community care' (Baldock and Ungerson, 1994) found that nearly all were offered at least 1 day a week at a day hospital. Whilst there, many received speech and language therapy or physiotherapy but: 'Speech therapy was what many were hoping for but not getting' (p. 19). If they tried to ask for a particular service: 'Usually they would receive no clear answer or would be told what they were asking for was not possible' (p. 19). Waiting lists, found in many speech and language therapy departments, indicate that demand exceeds supply. There is also anecdotal evidence (e.g. Law and Paterson, 1980; Edelman and Greenwood, 1992; ADA audiocassette, 1995) that many aphasic people value speech and language therapy highly. Certainly, many work extremely hard at their language over a protracted period. In relation to disabled people more generally, Silburn (1994) suggests that 'it is questionable to what extent people would want to be rehabilitated if they lived in a world where the struggle to learn to walk a few yards on crutches was made pointless by decent wheelchairs and a barrier-free environment' (p. 255). Experiences of living with aphasia described in Chapter 2 show that we are a very long way from a barrier-free society in relation to communication.

This is, however, most unlikely to be the whole story, given the centrality not just of communication but of conversation in our lives. Since conversation is concerned not only with the exchange of information (a major function in its own right) but also with self-definition (Kagan, 1995), losing the ability to converse freely is commonly experienced as a devastating psychological assault. By virtue of their technical knowledge, aphasia therapists offer aphasic people their best chance of maximizing both language and other communication skills. One-to-one therapy aiming to address language deficits and to improve functional communication is likely to remain the core of their work for the foreseeable future. In many instances it is not so much the *content* of services that would need to change with the adoption of the social model, as the *relationship* between the service provider and the aphasic person.

Treatment will be preceded by diagnostic testing. This is likely to be stressful for the aphasic person, since its purpose is to assess as specifically as possible where their speech and language problems lie, and hence to provide the therapist with information required before ways to help can be suggested. Furthermore, no immediate improvement for the aphasic person is anticipated from the assessment. The testing process will tend to place the therapist in a position of control, possibly making it difficult to avoid setting up the relationship as an unequal one in which the real power rests with the therapist.

The shift in location of services from hospital to community settings may have implications for the power of aphasic people compared with that of therapists. Aphasic people may feel more powerful because they are on their home ground – or at least in a setting not so associated with professional power as are hospitals. We must be careful not to overstate this possible effect, however. The attitudes, words and actions of aphasia therapists are likely to have a major influence here, whatever the setting. Focusing on the impairment may lead to negative stereotyping of aphasic people. Pound (1993) investigated attitudes of aphasic people and their therapists to the aphasia. Whilst difficulties were acknowledged, the aphasic people interviewed were aware that there could be benefits too (see also Chapter 2). Examples of benefits identified by aphasic people were a perceived change in their own temperament, which was hence associated with the ability to care more for other people. A number of those interviewed were enjoying the company of new friends or having increased time to pursue new leisure activities. A small number said that they felt happier and healthier following the stroke. Being aphasic had changed peoples' outlook on life in a variety of directions, whereas the speech and language therapists interviewed for the study assumed that becoming aphasic was a largely negative experience. Pound concludes that if therapists hold a negative attitude to disability it impedes the potential of aphasic people to take more control over their response to the consequences of the stroke in their lives. This calls for a critical approach by all aphasia therapists to their own attitudes and behaviour, in order to ensure that their practice breaks down disabling barriers wherever possible. Greater awareness of the multi-faceted nature of individuals' responses to impairment should foster more positive attitudes among professionals.

We commented at the end of Chapter 5 on the continued use of the term 'patient' in those parts of the health service concerned with the rehabilitation of people who are not 'ill' but who need services such as the various therapies to ameliorate the effects of impairment. The label has symbolic significance, implying a medical framework based on individual pathology and a quasimedical status for therapists. This is beginning to change. For example, the (then) CSLT standards document, *Communicating Quality* (1991) adopts the epithet 'client'. To embrace the social model fully, speech and language therapists will have to learn to perceive their clients in a more neutral way, perhaps simply as 'service users'.

In the community there are likely to be more players, and this immediately makes for a more complex distribution of power. In particular, there will probably be greater interaction between therapist and carer; indeed, the opportunity to see a partner or carer is commonly cited by therapists as one of the advantages of visiting a patient at home. As we pointed out in Chapter 4, carers have their own needs and interests. These may or may not coincide or be compatible with the aphasic person's, depending on the specific situation at issue. The aphasic person's and carer's separate needs must be distinguished in order to avoid confusion as to who the service is for. Our discussion of aphasia services in Chapter 5 makes it clear that speech and language therapists see themselves as providing a service for relatives as well as for aphasic people. Empowerment requires clarity as to existing distributions of power and *who* is to be empowered. Speech and language therapists need to be clear that *their primary responsibility is to the language-impaired person.*

What then is the nature of speech and language therapists' relationship with carers? Twigg's typology (1989) of agencies' perceptions of informal carers is instructive. She suggests that carers may be perceived as **resources**, **co-workers** or **co-clients**. Twigg and Atkin (1994) add a fourth category: the **superseded carer**. Viewed as resources by speech and language therapists, carers might be expected to provide therapy practice. This is typically a manager's perspective. The carer's own needs are disregarded under this model and it is assumed that there are no conflicts of interest between the disabled person and carer. Seeing carers as **co-workers**, or partners in providing a service, is a more usual perspective among front-line staff. There, there is some acknowledgement of the carers' own needs, but only in so far as these affect their ability to maximize the disabled person's welfare. A service for carers of aphasic people under this model might aim to improve carer morale so that the aphasic person would not be depressed and hence unable to benefit from aphasia therapy. Is this the rationale for some stroke relatives' support groups? The underlying assumption is that carers do want to care, and that the agencies' role should be to assist them in this self-imposed task. In other words, carers are expected to sacrifice their own needs for the good of the disabled person. We give our own view of such a stance in Chapter 9. Agencies have a vested interest in defining informal carers as widely as possible within both these models, in order to maximize assistance and thereby minimize their own necessary input.

If carers are viewed as **co-clients** then services may be provided for them in their own right, aiming to ease the burden of caring, and thus to improve the carer's welfare. This might be at the expense of the disabled person, at least in the short term. For example, it is possible to envisage a relative diverting an aphasia therapist into a discussion of communication difficulties from the carer's viewpoint when the plan had been to work with the aphasic person. It may be appropriate for the therapist to allow her or his time to be taken up in this way, if that appears to be in the aphasic person's longer-term interest. What is required is a conscious decision on the therapist's part together with the provision of clear information to the carer and, where possible, advice as to how the carer might take steps to meet his or her own needs. It may well be that the 'felt need' among therapists to provide relatives' support groups stems partly from the type of incident described above.

Finally, agencies may aim to **supersede** particular carers, either to relieve them from the burden of the carer role, or to empower the disabled person by promoting his or her independence. The latter may be applicable, in a limited way, in relation to aphasia. Several studies have typified some relatives as 'overprotective' (Malone, Ptacek and Malone, 1970; Mykyta *et al.*, 1976; Kinsella and Duffy, 1980; Chapter 2). The negative overtones of this description are unhelpful, but the message that some close relationships are not conducive to meeting an aphasic person's needs for opportunities to use language is, nevertheless, important. We touched on this earlier in this chapter in discussing 'disability level' practice. The aphasia therapist may encourage an aphasic person to participate in activities outside the confines and safety of their home perhaps through attending a group or with a volunteer, as described above (Lyon, 1989). It is worth noting that superseding carers for the disabled person's benefit will always have the side-effect of reducing the carer's responsibility. Such 'positive sum' strategies should be pursued whenever feasible.

We suggested in Chapter 5 that contracts between therapists and aphasic people could provide a framework for the construction of shared goals and negotiated treatment plans. Whilst contracts are possible with all patients, the contribution of the latter to contract delineation will vary. Writing about aphasia services in Belgium, where legal (i.e. compulsory) insurance covers up to four 6-month contracts for aphasia therapy, Seron and de Partz (1993) comment on aphasic people's increasing control over the content of their treatment. In negotiating the first contract, patients 'are very dependent on the suggestions of the therapist and accept almost all propositions presented to them' (p. 133). Later on, when patients have a clearer idea of their disability 'objectives become progressively more personalized and more related to the difficulties encountered by the patients in daily-life situations.' They give as an example a short contract aiming to enable an aphasic man 'to propose a toast at his daughter's wedding'.

Enabling an aphasic person whose understanding is badly affected to enter into the partnership implied by a contracting approach presents a particular challenge. Marsh and Fisher (1992) explore a comparable situation, though in relation to a different service and client group. Their discussion concerns the potential of a partnership model for social work interventions, and they consider how far this is possible for dementia sufferers. They conclude that 'a partnership *approach* can be used at all times, but it may not always lead directly to partnership *practice* for a limited number of cases concerning people with dementia' (p. 17, italics in the original). In relation to aphasic people whose understanding is severely impaired, the speech and language therapist will need to be sensitive to whatever clues are available as to the person's wishes. Marsh and Fisher state that 'maintaining involvement despite lack of consent substantially compromises the partnership principle' (p. 17). Aphasia therapy depends on the aphasic person's co-operation and, as we saw in Chapters 4 and 5, motivation is an important criterion in selection for active treatment. So any speech and language therapy input offered without the aphasic person's active consent is likely to be indirect. It might involve, for example, the provision of guidance to a carer. Here, it is essential that sight is not lost of the aim of reducing barriers for the aphasic person, who is the primary client.

SCARCE RESOURCES AND APHASIA THERAPY

Speech and language therapists' professional role requires them to ration their own time and also facilities such as accommodation and transport. For some therapists working in a stroke or rehabilitation unit caseloads may be kept relatively steady by the unit's admission policy. More usually, therapists do their own rationing. This often means coping with a variable rate of referral and workload. One method of managing excess demand is to target therapy towards those aphasic people who are expected to reap the greatest rewards from the attention. This method requires attention to the aims of any therapeutic activity, and continual re-evaluation with the aphasic person and carer of whether aims are being achieved. It also requires skilled management of aphasic people's and carers' expectations, coupled with the ability to give the former the confidence to feel that they can continue to recover without a long dependency on the therapist. It is important that people not selected for active treatment are reviewed periodically so that they have the opportunity to receive therapy later on if appropriate.

Another method of rationing services is to modify quality standards. So, for example, maximum response times to referrals may be extended from 5 days to 10 days, or the service may be able to offer only assessment and advice but not active treatment. We explained in Chapter 5 that some departments use working with groups as a way of rationing scarce resources. The adult service manager in one department in our 'pathways' study (Kaiser and Jordan, unpublished report) was planning to meet 'continuing care' needs through voluntary organizations and a self-help group so as to utilize professional speech and language therapy skills as efficiently as possible. As suggested earlier, great care is required to ensure that aphasic people's needs are kept to the forefront in such policies. Departments' decisions about rationing within aphasia services should be concerned with assessing the relative benefits to aphasic people of, for example:

- rapidity of response;
- individual and group therapy;

- different degrees of commitment to the 'continuing care' of aphasic people (e.g. how active a role speech and language therapists should be playing in 'speech after stroke' clubs and liaison with adult education services for aphasic people);
- investing in community education, as in 'shop sign' projects (described in Chapter 9);
- applying for research and development monies.

Speech and language therapy departments' decisions about the priorities to put forward in contract negotiations will probably be taken in the context of adult services as a whole, or even across the board (that is, alongside services for children). There will be exceptions here. For example, speech and language therapist staffing for a new stroke unit would almost certainly be accorded priority at all levels. Current service patterns in particular localities may depend to a considerable extent on historical factors (Jordan, 1991; Kaiser and Jordan, unpublished data). Existing patterns may be protected by powerful hidden assumptions, for example that the current distribution of resources among different client groups is 'about right'. Arguably, decisions on this matter should belong to the political realm rather than being seen as technical matters for professional judgement. We do know that considerable variations have been found in the percentage of total speech and language therapy service hours devoted to services for adults (Rossiter and McInally, 1989). Staffing therefore depends more on funding than on need. Decisions about future funding usually take current provision as their main point of reference, though there is at least the potential for a more radical approach to be built into contracting within a quasi-market system.

The introduction of quasi-markets in the NHS is forcing health services to operate more like private sector businesses. If individual services are to compete successfully for health resources, they must define their 'product' and actively market it. It is important that the results of rationing decisions being made within a provider organization are fed back to purchasers, together with information on how standards of service in the area concerned compare with those recommended by the RCSLT and with standards in other areas. In Chapters 3 and 6 we referred to the absence of satisfactory information about the incidence and prevalence of aphasia, both nationally and in most localities. This needs to be remedied by the collection and collation of reliable data into local stroke registers. Diagnosis by speech and language therapists is essential here.

'Front-line' speech and language therapists have the privilege of access to information about aphasic people's needs and preferences. We would argue that their professional responsibility includes being alert to the implications of such information in terms of service provision. This might mean the identification of gaps in provision, or of practices that create barriers for aphasic people or do little to remove such barriers. What is required is a research orientation, which in this context means:

- mentally collating and interpreting information;
- checking out interpretations with service users;
- sharing hunches with colleagues in their own geographical areas and further afield (through involvement in professional specific-interest groups and activities of the British Aphasiology Society, for example);
- participating in debate about future provision, including discussion about how and by whom it can most appropriately be organized;
- being prepared to put forward a case for additional resources or for changing procedures in order to improve the use of existing resources.

The most suitable forum for debate will vary, as will the most appropriate channel through which to present such a case. One avenue is likely to be through managers within the employing service and via them to purchasers. Another route is via publication in professional newsletters or journals. It may often be most productive to pursue as many different channels as possible.

Health services in Britain have to operate within tight financial constraints, so arguing for an increase in resources for a particular service could be seen as risking credibility. Given the gross shortfalls in staffing these services have compared with what is needed (e.g. Enderby and Davies, 1989) we would argue that, on the contrary, we could not retain credibility if we failed to put forward such an argument. That inadequate speech and language therapy staffing is widely acknowledged is suggested by the fact that, when asked to evaluate the experimental employment of speech and language therapy assistants, the main concern expressed by members of other professions (teaching, occupational therapy, physiotherapy, management, etc.) 'was that there continued to be a shortfall of speech and language therapy provision, even with the deployment of speech and language assistants' (Davies and van der Gaag, 1993).

Rationing within a social model framework demands that priorities are set in line with service users' self-defined needs and preferences, rather than by reference to professional assumptions. At the level of individual practice, treating service users as equals (a prerequisite for their empowerment) requires openness and clarity about resource restrictions and rationing decisions. Ellis (1993), writing about community care assessment, acknowledges the tensions this can create between front-line staff and managers. She nevertheless suggests that:

making the process of resource management explicit provides opportunities as well as challenges. Not only competing but also common
interests may be revealed, paving the way for alliances to be forged
between different interest groups – to fight for more resources for
example.

(p. 40)

Drawing aphasic people themselves into debates about resourcing and
priorities may enable a more powerful case to be made. It should also ensure
that priorities more closely reflect relevance to aphasic people, thus fostering
effectiveness and value for money.

ASSURING QUALITY

Speech and language therapists have, over many years, been prepared to
look critically at different ways of working in order to establish best
practice, and the profession has been at the forefront in developing quality
standards (CST Aphasia Working Party, 1989; CSLT, 1991). Clinical audit
is also established in many if not all speech and language therapy departments (e.g. Enderby, 1992; Barnett, 1994; Fielden, 1994; Hull and Wilson,
1994).

A social model framework implies demanding audit requirements. This
is because tools have not been developed to measure the extent to which
social barriers are overcome. The theoretical and methodological difficulties in devising appropriate outcome measures should not be underestimated; most service evaluation utilizes input and output measures rather
than measures of outcome. A qualitative approach may be more effective in
capturing the 'essence' of outcome, but this would increase the cost of
auditing.

The quality of a service is bound to be affected by the degree of expertise
and experience of its staff. The interests of aphasic people are best served
by access to experienced specialist staff, but the organization of speech and
language therapy and career structures within the speech and language therapy profession tend to mitigate against this. Many specialist posts that
include aphasia are in neurology, a much broader area not confined to language work. Especially in relatively poorly staffed services, therapists nom-
inally in specialist posts may be expected to undertake a wider range of
cases than is indicated by their job title.

Junior posts recruiting newly qualified therapists are usually generalist.
It is argued that attaining experience in relation to a wide range of disorders
is necessary to enable therapists to make informed choices about subsequent specialization. Rossiter (1987) put forward the idea of rotational

posts, whereby incumbents would spend (say) 6 months in each of a range of specialisms. Rossiter argued that rotational posts would enable the speech and language therapy profession to maintain a higher profile because each therapist would be covering a smaller number of sites during the week, but another advantage would be to allow the therapist to work intensively on a relatively narrow range of cases during each block of time, thus rapidly building up expertise. Close and specialist supervision is likely to be facilitated, thus aiding skills development in newly qualified staff. In one urban area with several junior staff where rotational posts have been tried, they have been found to work extremely well. They broadened the range of experiences for rotational staff and meant that local therapists were available to fill specialist posts when they arose. They encouraged the whole service to develop supportive strategies and induction packs for new entrants. However, pressures under the contacting system and reduced movement of staff have unfortunately led to the discontinuance of this scheme.

Specialist posts are higher graded and recruit therapists with at least a few years of clinical experience. For a proportion of speech and language therapists, specialization is a career stage. Further promotion means managerial responsibilities, and a reduction in or the cessation of clinical work. This means that some of the most experienced (and most prominent) clinical specialists are continually being lost from clinical practice. Former aphasia specialists in management are, however, arguably in a stronger position to influence decisions and thus to protect aphasia services.

WORKING FOR STAFF AS WELL AS FOR PATIENTS?

An underlying assumption of *Working for Patients*, the policy document heralding the introduction of quasi-markets in the NHS (DoH, 1989b; also Chapter 6), was that services had hitherto been organized more for the convenience of staff than in patients' interests. The ensuing policy sought to establish the primacy of patients' needs. One consequent danger was that staff would feel devalued. As stated in Chapter 6, NHS staff have had to cope with the recurrent uncertainties that inevitably accompany a prolonged period of rapid organizational change and to come to terms with a new culture that promotes competition among provider units rather than co-operation.

Staff welfare and morale are issues that all employers should take seriously. They are important goals in their own right. They are also important on instrumental grounds since:

- dissatisfaction leads to high drop-out rates. A recent study found a 25% loss at 12 years post-qualification, with half the leavers in other areas of

employment, representing 'a huge loss in financial terms as well as in lost experience and expertise' (RCSLT Bulletin, 1995b, p. 1);
• demoralized staff are most unlikely to be able to give of their best.

Having staff who feel highly valued is particularly crucial where the aim is to empower service users, rather than simply to offer them a service. As Stevenson and Parsloe (1993) state: 'If users are to be empowered they need empowered staff. This ... means staff who are imaginative, enthusiastic, realistic, knowledgeable and justly confident' (p. 48). We consider two aspects here, namely speech and language therapy education and factors making for a supportive environment for therapists in post.

Speech and language therapy education

The training of speech and language therapists for work with aphasic people has some common themes across Britain, such as teaching theoretical bases for assessment and direct treatment of aspects of aphasia. Training on the clinical application of any theory is undertaken largely by independent clinical supervisors in the field and with widely varying degrees of integration with course content. For example, some undergraduate training courses require clinical supervisors to attend training on supervision and provide supervisors with detailed feedback from students following each placement. Others simply give a copy of the course syllabus, expecting clinicians to be able to impart their own understanding of how theory and practice interrelate for the benefit of the aphasic person. This factor may to some extent account for the wide variation in the appreciation by newly qualified clinicians of their role in aphasia, based as it is partly on academic learning and partly on observations and experience attained during clinical placements. *Communicating Quality* (CSLT, 1991) gives broad guidelines on the role of speech and language therapists with aphasic people, but does not go beyond recommending that therapists consider the patient as a whole.

The content of academic courses varies from institution to institution though many courses leading to professional qualification in speech and language therapy have a heavy psychological bias. The shift from hospital to community locations for speech and language therapy calls for expansion of this theoretical base to one more broadly based in social science. New areas for research, such as conversational analysis and therapy, necessitate shifts in a similar direction. Kagan and Gailey (1993) conclude from their discussion of the North York Aphasia Centre's work: 'We anticipate that the study of conversation will become as necessary a part of the speech–language pathology curriculum as the study of language is today' (p. 220).

Finkelstein (1991) suggests that we should be 'improving the education and training of community based service providers so that their analytical and organisational skills are better focussed on barrier identification and removal' (p. 37).

In order to establish the social model of disability as the fundamental basis for speech and language therapy practice it is essential that under-graduates are exposed to ideas about concepts of disability. They need to examine both the underlying values of models of disability and their application to aphasia therapy. Kagan's seminal article 'Revealing the competence of aphasic adults through conversation: a challenge to health professionals' (1995) should be classed as essential reading for all speech and language therapy students. 'High quality disability equality training' is also called for (French, 1994b, p. 111). At least some courses are already addressing such issues. However, there is a need for their incorporation into the curriculum at both undergraduate and postgraduate levels and for short courses and workshops to update clinicians throughout the country.

Creating a supportive working environment

Sharing with colleagues any ideas about what can best help a particular language-impaired person may be helpful even for experienced clinicians, and easy access to clinical supervision and advice is essential for the less experienced. The national survey of Mackenzie *et al.* (1993; Chapter 5, p. 70) found that supervision was available to most, but not all, therapists in the lowest-graded posts, but to only a minority of more senior staff.

Support in relation to clinical decisions may be achieved in different ways. Managers can ensure that the departmental culture fosters open exchange of ideas by making this an explicit expectation. The allocation of responsibilities for the supervision of junior staff needs to be clear to all. It may be possible to set up situations to enable therapists to develop confidence in one another and provide peer support. For example, one service in our 'pathways' study (Kaiser and Jordan, unpublished report; Chapter 5) deploys staff in such a way that no therapist is isolated on one site. This does have an impact on patient care, in that inpatients might be seen (for monitoring, advice and support) by up to three therapists. Elsewhere, clinicians might work together to run a therapy group, thereby also providing opportunities for mutual support. Staff support groups are another idea. Patch systems are often associated with isolation of staff, that is, if one member of staff covers each service location. Isolation of therapists is often a particular problem in rural areas, and strategies are required to counter-act this.

Postgraduate education, activities run by national organizations such as the British Aphasiology Society and the RCSLT and meetings of local specific-interest groups afford opportunities to raise and discuss clinical issues with other aphasia therapists. About 80% of aphasia therapists responding to the national survey mentioned above had the chance to undertake postgraduate education, and a similar percentage reported access to meetings with aphasia colleagues. Half the respondents had opportunities to conduct research.

It must be recognized that certain aspects of work in relation to aphasia are particularly challenging. A recently qualified therapist commented to one of the authors that working with individual patients was hard enough, so she certainly did not feel ready to contemplate trying to manage a group. Younger therapists might also be expected to find supporting relatives difficult, partly, no doubt, due to their limited life experience and difficulties in attaining and maintaining credibility with some relatives who may prejudge them by their comparative youth. Similar problems may occur with aphasic people themselves. Managers need to be explicit about what should be expected of newly qualified speech and language therapists who, in turn, need to be clear about how much they should expect of themselves.

In Chapter 6 we discussed some of the pressures arising from the environment within which speech and language therapy departments operate. There would seem to be a lack of congruence between organizational requirements and the needs of the language-impaired clientele. Speech and language therapy's location in the NHS means that certain kinds of service developments are favoured and others are unlikely to be considered, let alone accepted. Contractors demand proof of value for money, efficiency and effectiveness, and this leads to an emphasis on the production of statistical data to give numerical measures of performance. This contrasts oddly with the 'softer' (but arguably at least as important) aims of much aphasia therapy. There is a real danger of the most important aspects of what aphasic people achieve with the assistance of speech and language therapists being discounted because they are not reducible to a few figures on a spreadsheet. Identifying an inherent conflict between therapeutic goals on the one hand and what is required as health authority activity information on the other is likely to cause feelings of dissonance in therapists.

The NHS's strong organizational and professional boundaries can be comfortably protective at times, but they can also constrain therapists into providing 'standard' services, which may not be the best thing for all patients. Many speech and language therapists work in acute hospital settings where a medical model of care reigns supreme. Yet they are often closely involved with aphasic people and their families, aware of both the unmet needs and that the knowledge they (therapists) hold could enable them to help the aphasic person through some of the main consequences of the stroke. Speech and language therapists may also become aware at times that the role in which they were trained is not always appropriately applied for some aphasic people, or that they require support in areas in which the speech and language therapist would not traditionally respond. In this situation the therapist is faced with different and conflicting demands, stemming on the one hand from professional expectations and the confines of the NHS and on the other from either observation of the aphasic person or (ideally) that person's self-expressed needs. If the social model is to be operationalized, professional and organizational obligations have to be eased sufficiently to provide whatever flexibility is required by aphasic people's needs for services.

As speech and language therapy moves out into the community, there will be new pressures on staff, but also new opportunities. Speech and language therapists are likely to find themselves working more closely than hitherto with local authority social services, where social model ideas are more prevalent than in the NHS. In our view, the values of the speech and language therapy profession are not incompatible with the social model of disability, though fully embracing it would require some major adjustments in thinking. At least in the short to medium term, we might expect greater exposure to social model thinking among front-line workers to lead to increased tensions first between therapists and their managers and then between speech and language therapy departments and other parts of the NHS. The degree of tension will depend to some extent on the impact of the social model elsewhere in the NHS. Adoption of the social model may also mean discrepancy between what therapists are trained to do and what they find themselves doing. At the same time, speech and language therapists may experience greater congruence between what they can offer and aphasic people's needs. There is evidence that social model ways of working lead to professionals being very highly valued by service users. Lonsdale (1990) comments on the 'gratitude, enthusiasm and warmth' of the disabled women she interviewed towards health professionals who were 'helpful and acted in partnership with them' (p. 52).

RESEARCH

The decade from 1985 to 1995 has been characterized by an explosion of theoretical insights at the impairment level and the incorporation of some of these ideas into day-to-day practice. The field of cognitive neuropsychology (Chapter 3, p. 43) has been particularly fruitful. There is no doubt that greater precision in therapists' understanding of individuals' language deficits and ability to treat these are in the interests of aphasic people as a group but, as Parr, Pound and Marshall (1995) suggest: 'Scientific, highly theoretical therapy programmes run the risk of exciting and empowering the therapist, whilst failing to engage the aphasic person in a more equal relationship' (p. 9). Conversation analysis (Chapter 4, p. 59) runs the same risks. It is concerned with the transference of **meaning** within aphasic conversation, and is thus a tool for conversational 'ramping'. Nevertheless, to most aphasic people it is likely to appear an exotic and impenetrable technique. It may be only marginally less so to aphasia therapists.

Clarity of thought and openness with aphasic people are required about the likely costs and benefits to them of their participation in research studies. Testing and retesting of 'subjects' may be a necessary part of research protocol but is unlikely to have relevance in the lives of the aphasic people involved. Where the potential benefits to aphasic 'subjects' themselves are slight, consideration should be given to paying them for their contribution. Many aphasic people might be happy to participate in research to benefit other aphasic people on an unpaid basis. According them the status of 'volunteer' and paying their expenses would avoid the risk of exploitation.

Social model thinking brings with it a new research agenda for speech and language therapists, together with a commitment to the active involvement of aphasic people in the decision-making process. Parr and Gilpin (1995) describe the pioneering role here of one project. Issues relating to social structural factors such as class, gender and ethnicity are yet to be explored in relation to aphasia. There will also be a need to evaluate new ways of working.

The interaction of research with practice and aphasic people's role in sparking the development of research ideas are illustrated in the work of the North York Aphasia Centre. Kagan and Gailey (1993) emphasize that their approach:

> originates directly from our observation of interactions of chronic aphasic individuals and trained volunteers who participate in the Centre's programs. Shifts in professional focus are, therefore, as much the result of lessons aphasic adults and volunteers have taught us as they are of changing perspectives in the field of speech–language pathology. Current theory and research in the area of conversation provide an explanatory framework for a process that has developed spontaneously.
>
> *(p. 200)*

The coming years promise to be a challenging and exciting time for aphasia research. In order to rise to the challenge, researchers will need humility, imagination and a willingness to question received ideas about aphasia therapy and the speech and language therapist's professional role.

9 | Quality of life with aphasia: towards empowerment

In Chapter 2 people affected by aphasia described their lives, showing both what a devastating disability aphasia can be and the capacity of many people affected by it to find and enjoy a new way of life. In subsequent chapters we have explained, in so far as is possible, the nature of aphasia and considered the main services with which aphasic people are likely to come into contact. Chapter 8 explored some parameters for the practice of aphasia therapy based on the social model of disability. It is now time to turn once again to aphasic people's lives as a whole. Our aim in this final chapter is to identify strategies that can help maintain or improve the quality of aphasic people's experience of life across the whole spectrum. Our discussion is necessarily wide ranging, reflecting the number and diversity of factors that impinge on quality of life.

We start with a brief analysis of two key concepts used in the chapter, **quality of life** and **empowerment**, showing how these concepts relate to each other. The rest of the chapter is structured in terms of the roles of aphasic people at three levels: as individuals, in their interactions with service organizations and in relation to society. At the 'individual' level, we consider the potential for improving quality of aphasic life in different arenas. At the 'organizational' level we outline three models for the distribution of decision-making power between the organization and its clientele and illustrate the application of each in relation to aphasic people and organizations with which they are concerned. Finally, we consider the position of aphasia and aphasic people in society. To date, this can best be described as a 'non-position', since aphasia goes largely unheard of, unrecognized and little understood. We identify the beginnings of change and then suggest strategies for spreading the word about aphasia.

DEFINING QUALITY OF LIFE AND EMPOWERMENT

Non-disabled people often see quality of life for disabled people in terms of **independence**. This implies being able to look after yourself, live in your own home, perhaps earn your own living, get to places like shops and banks, and use them. Whilst independence is undoubtedly relevant to quality of life, it would be wrong to assume that it is the main goal for disabled people. In practice, ordinary life involves **interdependence**; in modern industrial societies complete self-reliance is virtually unknown. Typically, there is a division of labour whereby, for example, certain members of a household may regularly undertake particular tasks like shopping, making social arrangements or letter writing (Parr, 1995). The ways in which we depend on others vary according to many factors of which disability is just one but, as French (1993b) suggests, disability-related dependency is commonly perceived as problematic. French challenges this perception. She argues that: 'giving and receiving help can greatly enrich human experience' and that:

> Narrowly defined, independence can give rise to inefficiency, stress and isolation, as well as wasting precious time. Striving for independence ... can lead to frustration and low self-esteem ... An over-emphasis on physical independence can rob disabled people of true independence by restricting their freedom of thought and action
>
> *(p. 47)*

Disabled people agree that the key factor is the **ability to control their own lives**. This means making your own decisions, ranging from ones involving minor day-to-day activities (e.g. when to have a bath, phone a friend), through ones affecting an aspect of your life in the short to medium term (e.g. whether to participate in an outing, join a club) to decisions about major, perhaps long-term, directions to take (e.g. where to live or work, whether to retire, whether to let someone else take some decisions for you). Of course, having a free choice is unusual. Another member of your household may be in the bath or using the phone, or your friend may be out. You may lack the time, enthusiasm and/or money to become involved in a particular social commitment. The major decisions are likely to be constrained above all by your income, but also by other factors such as potential employers' requirements and their perceptions of you, and the needs and wishes of other members of your family. The defining feature of 'independent living' is thus **control over decisions** rather than performance by the disabled person of particular tasks or activities.

This perspective on independent living has implications for disabled people's own goals and for the aims of rehabilitation. For disabled people, it means that learning not to put all your energy into attempting to remaster tasks that have now become too difficult is a valid aim that can in itself be seen as a skill (Anderson, 1992). For rehabilitation, it means a shift of emphasis towards helping disabled people to be realistic and relaxed in their own decisions about what they can reasonably do, supporting them in decisions to stop trying so hard to do the mundane and together applying creative lateral thinking about alternative ways to achieve their goals without thereby burdening their families.[1] The challenge of this agenda should not be underestimated; 'giving up' has such negative connotations in our society that it is likely to be difficult for many disabled people to see it as the positive step it can sometimes be. To the extent that 'personality changes' after stroke reported by some carers (Anderson, 1992) stem from the frustrations of life with impairment rather than from the insult to the brain, we might expect this approach to make for a reduction in stress for the disabled person and therefore to ease relationships.

Control over decision making equals power, a concept we discussed briefly in Chapter 1. We are concerned in this chapter with exploring strategies to effect a redistribution of power in the direction of aphasic people: in short, their empowerment. Empowerment has been something of a buzzword in the first half of the 1990s, and is seriously at risk of being 'all things to all people' and thus becoming a meaningless platitude. There is an inherent difficulty in avoiding such a danger in that, arguably, power is a factor in all human relationships. It follows that the potential for empowerment (or, conversely, for reinforcing powerlessness) is very pervasive. We use a wide range of examples, ranging from the minutae of day-to-day life to cultural change, to explore how aphasic people might be empowered. Whilst we aim to provide some benchmarks, our approach is discursive rather than prescriptive.

In order to sharpen the focus on empowerment, it is useful to summarize some of the things about aphasia that disable, disadvantage and disempower aphasic people. First there is the impairment itself. The centrality of language means that the inability to use it easily, accurately and fluently has implications for all aspects of life. Severe aphasia impairs and dislocates relationships. Even mild aphasia can be experienced as an appreciable disability, perhaps entailing problems in maintaining established domestic, employment and leisure roles, leading to loss of confidence and self-esteem. As explained in Chapter 1, the social model sees the source of disability as lying outside the individual. We have argued throughout this book that the social model offers a new – and better – way of thinking about aphasia and responding to aphasic people. Nevertheless, aphasia imposes specific limitations that in themselves make life more difficult for the aphasic person. By virtue of this burden, aphasia tends to disempower people.

The limitations imposed by aphasia are compounded by major factors external to the aphasic person. First, aphasic people are disabled by attitudes towards them. Block and Yuker (1979) suggest that effecting changes in attitudes towards disability is the key to improving disabled people's life chances. It is arguable that attitudes take on an added importance in relation to aphasia because language, one of the principal means by which attitudes are conveyed, is at the heart of the impairment. Aphasia is not apparent to others until the aphasic person tries to communicate, and this may make the disorder less readily comprehensible than more visible impairments such as paralysis. So aphasic people often meet with bewilderment, uncertainty and embarrassment from other people. Block and Yuker summarize research findings that suggest that some impairments elicit more negative attitudes than others and in particular that: 'The most rejected persons are those with the most non-normal appearance or behaviour which may be hard to ignore. Thus facial disfigurement, *brain damage involving strange speech patterns* or strange gait are hard for people to adjust to' (p. 2, emphasis added).

Next, aphasic people may be disadvantaged by what the (then) CST Aphasia Working Party (1989) termed 'reduced lobbying power ... by virtue of their handicap' (p. 7). Whilst being aphasic undoubtedly makes it more difficult for people to advance their own cause, there is ample evidence to show that it does not necessarily make it impossible (Chapter 2; City Dysphasic Group, 1989; Edelman and Greenwood, 1992). We must also question to what extent the difficulties result from negative attitudes, rather than from the disorder *per se.*

Finally, aphasic adults suffer, at least in Britain, from 'the lack of sufficiently strong advocacy' (CST Aphasia Working Party 1989, p. 7). Advocacy may be for an individual or for a group. We have discussed self-advocacy to some extent in the last paragraph. There are several reasons for the low profile of aphasia as a cause. Speech and language therapists, the professionals most closely involved with aphasic people, are not a powerful group within the NHS and not all speech and language therapists see aphasia services as a high priority (ibid). Furthermore, aphasic people form a minority of the stroke population and it is arguable that communication impairment is given less emphasis by the medical profession than, for example, mobility. (Whilst medical attention may itself be disabling and disempowering (Illich, 1976; Lonsdale, 1990; Barnes, 1991, Chapter 6), inattention to communication disorder is no less so.) Many carers do not have the time or energy to do more than cope from day to day.

Advocacy may be provided by voluntary organizations. An international survey of organizations concerned with aphasia suggests that it is only comparatively recently that national organizations have been set up specifically for aphasia (Jordan, 1995b). Examples include ADA in the UK (founded in

1980), Japanese Peer Circles (1983), Federation Nationale des Aphasiques de France (1985) and the Aphasia National Association in the USA (1987). The survey elicited responses from five other specialist aphasia organizations, in Switzerland, Canada, Norway, Belgium and Italy, all of which had started between 1984 and 1994. Stroke organizations in some countries have a much longer history, though concern with aphasia seems to have increased during the 1970s and 1980s. The Association Internationale Aphasie (AIA) was created in Brussels in 1989 to bring together the growing number of national bodies. Whilst such organizations have considerable potential in advocacy, there is a limit to what can be achieved from a low base of public knowledge, often with very limited resources. We give examples of initiatives taken by aphasia organizations in a number of countries later in this chapter.

APHASIC INDIVIDUALS AND EMPOWERMENT

Here we focus on quality of life and empowerment in different locations where aphasic people – private households and residential settings – and in relation to different kinds of activity, namely social and 'everyday' activities and employment.

Living at home with aphasia

For the aphasic person living at home, the attitudes of other members of the household and how they attempt to cope with the disability are of considerable importance. Especially at first, a carer will probably be the aphasic person's main source of human contact, as well as of practical help and emotional support. One carer whose husband had very little speech made a point of getting him to choose between alternative menus rather than just presenting him with a meal. Being aphasic might, however, mean being unable to suggest a food you particularly fancy. Carers can, like Jim (Chapter 2, p. 16), insist that other people should speak directly to the aphasic person, and can at least check out any arrangement with him or her.

As we saw in Chapter 2, some people work very hard to help 'their' aphasic person to regain language skills. Every family is different, and what works for one family may be quite inappropriate in another. There are different views among professionals on how friends and relatives can best help. One speech and language therapist told us that she involves relatives and other carers in the same way that other therapists do volunteers. Others like to keep family members' and volunteers' roles distinct and separate. Examples here can be found in the practice of two of the projects discussed in Chapter 7. The Speakeasy Club does not accept members' relatives as volunteers. The Aphasia Centre – North York in Canada does accept relatives in this capacity, but is large enough to ensure that they are not in a group with their own aphasic person. The Centre has a clear policy in relation to members' families and friends. An information sheet (1994b) explains to them the distinction between providing opportunities for conversation on the one hand and improving communicative effectiveness on the other. It describes the speech–language pathologist's role in helping 'to improve verbal abilities' and helping aphasic people 'compensate for impaired verbal abilities by using effective non-verbal strategies', and the role of volunteers at the Centre 'in encouraging the use of these strategies and in providing opportunities for practice'. Its information sheet for families and friends continues:

> We do not recommend that you, as a family member or friend, assume this role. This is something we can do for you. The Speech–Language Pathology staff are more than willing to discuss and demonstrate the strategies we use so that you can focus on genuine conversation and interaction. This is what will make the most difference to your aphasic family member or friend because it enables you to re-establish your relationship with them.
>
> *(ibid.)*

The Centre also runs training and counselling sessions for families, and stresses the availability of staff to answer questions.

In any family, different members' needs and wishes sometimes conflict. For example, there may be pressure on the disabled person, from a carer desperately in need of a break, to attend a club or group. Not everyone wants to participate in communal activity. Adults in our society expect to make such decisions themselves, so to be told 'you'll enjoy it when you get there', or 'it'll be good for you', however true, tends to define someone out of their adult status.

Carers tend to be expected continually to put others' needs above their own (Dalley, 1988). We would argue that the disabled person's and carer's quality of life are equally important. This implies that the disabled person as well as the carer may have to make compromises. Some aphasic people realize, and are distressed by, the effects of their disability on their carers' lives (Mulhall, 1978). Others' conceptions of their carer's needs may differ from the carer's perception. In some instances carers' own fears and expectations may prevent them from acknowledging their needs to others, or even to themselves. This calls for accessible literature (e.g. Swaffield, 1990) and counselling to help all parties accept that it may benefit the disabled person for others' needs sometimes to come first, and to help work out ways round practical barriers. Possible benefits include improving the carer's quality of life, enabling the carer to cope or to cope better, and affirming the aphasic person's role as a responsible adult.

We have alluded to the need of aphasic people's relatives for support services, a need to which too little attention has been paid (Anderson, 1988). Slack and Mulville (1988) describe their attempts, not always successful, to obtain private help, in a book that illustrates carers' dilemmas, shows the dignity and 'quality of life' possible despite severe disability, and provides much practical advice for carers.

The Stroke Association has developed two services that are relevant here. Its community services division has set up a network of Stroke Information Centres throughout England and Wales. These offer a range of literature, a 'Listening Ear', and appropriate local contact points to stroke people and carers (Stroke Association, 1993c). There were 30 such centres by June 1995. The Stroke Association Community Services Family Support was operational in 28 health districts in England and Wales by the same date, and growing rapidly. This is a visiting service providing information, literature and emotional support for new stroke families. It runs on similar lines to Dysphasic Support (Chapter 5) with a Family Support Organizer who recruits volunteers. Family Support Organizers are health professionals and trained counsellors, and volunteers 'undertake a basic listening skills course and undergo training by the Organizer, other Stroke Association staff and relevant professionals' (Stroke Association, 1993b).

Relatives' or carers' groups have evolved in a number of areas, to provide information and support (Chapter 5). The impetus might come from a speech and language therapist, social worker or voluntary organization. One of the ADA aphasia self-help groups (discussed in a later section of this chapter) was set up by aphasic people who were already members of their local ADA branch precisely because they felt the branch was working as a group mainly for the benefit of carers. There is an important self-help element in all groups that allows relatives to meet others coping with similar difficulties. More specifically, a relatives' support group should provide a forum in which it is acceptable for carers to discuss both practical and emotional problems. Sharing 'negative' feelings, for example of frustration, anger and depression may reduce relatives' possible guilt and self-dislike at their reaction to changed circumstances, and/or to the disabled person's new self.

The potential for meeting carers' needs via a group is in our view rather limited. It may be an approach that is more popular with service providers than with carers themselves. We know of several attempts to establish carers' groups that have failed despite experimentation with different meeting times and formats. Practical difficulties for carers in attending are undoubtedly an important factor. It may be that service providers should be alert to any local demand for such groups rather than aiming to be proactive.

Group support for carers may happen as a spin-off from other aphasia or stroke-related activities. We have already noted that local ADA branches can serve this function and that some Stroke Association Dysphasic Support services hold regular or occasional meetings for carers (see Chapter 7). Otherwise, it may be that carers need individual attention from a speech and language therapist, a counsellor or another source they have sought out.

By no means all aphasic people need a carer, and many live on their own. Their situation is less complicated in that there is no close relative whose needs have to be considered. Responsibility for accessing opportunities for communication cannot so readily be shared and they might be seen as top priority where aftercare is limited. Living alone might be expected to affect someone's communication needs, but it is not possible to predict precisely how. For some aphasic people it might mean more need of group activities; others may prefer their own company. The communicative demands of day-to-day living are also likely to vary, with one person dealing with all her own affairs, whilst another has considerable amounts of help from informal and/or formal sources.

Access to everyday activities

Some attempts have been made to facilitate access to activities such as shopping for people with speech and language impairments. One example is a credit-card-style plastic identity card that indicates the nature of the holder's impairment. Such cards are offered by several charities, including ADA and The Stroke Association.

'Shop Sign' projects are an extension of this idea, coupling the use of identity cards with a shop window sign of the kind widely available for deaf people. What was probably the first such scheme in Britain was in Bury, Lancashire. The sign had to be simple but specific and the symbol used on ADA identity cards was chosen. 'Outlets' for the sign included local branches of chain stores, libraries, the Post Office, banks and building societies. They were offered written information (a simple list of points to remember when talking to speech-impaired people), stickers with the logo to put into windows, on checkouts, etc., and training for their staff in how to help people with speech impairments. Commenting on the advantages of the shop sign project, the speech and language therapist wrote:

> Our patients are far happier about shopping now. They all carry the ADA Identity Cards ... which they can use if in trouble. We have formed many valuable links with the local community, Marks and Spencer staff now fund raise regularly for us ... Libraries have become

involved in getting special books and cassettes to use in therapy sessions.

(Holland, S. unpublished report, Bury Health Authority c. 1987)

More recently, ADA Cambridge has embarked on a similar project.

In 1995 the Benefits Agency introduced a Basic Skills Help Scheme to assist social security claimants with communication or literacy problems in accessing appropriate assistance when visiting benefits offices. The scheme involves a credit-card-style card on which areas of difficulty can be indicated.

Access to transport for aphasic people may be facilitated by initiatives like London Regional Transport (LRT) notepads for people with impaired speech. These alerted bus crews to the passenger's problem, and had space for a note of the intended destination. Whilst free of charge, the notepads had to be obtained from the LRT Unit for Disabled Passengers (Cohen, 1987), so were not particularly accessible. Newcastle has a scheme whereby any communicatively impaired passenger can indicate that they would like to use a touchcard designed with the aid of speech and language therapists. The bus driver is trained to facilitate the use of the touchcard for the passenger to identify their destination and fare.

Employment

Employment can be an important symbol of achievement, as well as the means to income, social contacts and status. As we saw in Chapter 2, a minority of aphasic people do return to paid employment. We outlined employment services in Chapter 6. Here we consider some of the issues that arise and suggest factors to aid successful return to work.

In employment, we have to accept other people's assessment of our abilities and limitations. This contrasts markedly with the desirable emphasis in rehabilitation on building people's confidence in their ability to control their own lives. Despite being well aware of their dependence on potential or actual employers' decisions, aphasic people may require help to accept others' assessments of their abilities and, perhaps, extra assistance in the work setting. They may also benefit from the opportunity to practise employment-related skills. One of the ADA self-help groups held a mock job interview given by the local manager of a well-known international chain store.

To enable successful return to work, co-operation between those involved will be necessary. This includes not only the aphasic person and employer, but also perhaps an occupational therapist, speech and language therapist, disability employment adviser and coworkers. The employer will need information in order to make a realistic assessment of what can be expected of the aphasic employee. This will inform the employer's decision as to whether to (re)employ the aphasic person, and whether or not employment in a similar capacity as before is realistic. Downgrading may be particularly difficult to accept for someone returning to work with the same employer, but this may be his or her best chance of obtaining employment. This situation calls for much sensitivity on the part of employers and coworkers, and perhaps counselling for the aphasic person.

The return to work itself may need to be carefully planned, with coworkers being provided with information about aphasia. Flexibility may well be important. The employer might agree to conditions such as shorter hours and alternative work for an induction period. One school-teacher was able to work in the school library and sit in on classes, initially for only 1 or 2 days a week. The aphasic person may need to retrain, and also to accept his or her limitations. One young aphasic man was so keen that he worked every day even though his contract was for only 3 days a week. He 'burnt himself out' and became unemployed.

With increasing acceptance of the social model of disability, opportunities for employment in the 'aphasia industry' are opening up for small numbers of the most able and well-qualified aphasic people. Such aphasic people are beginning to become involved in several areas, notably counselling of other aphasic people and their families, lecturing and research. Providing such opportunities for aphasic people is a way of giving them status and, at least indirectly, greater visibility. It can be an important form of barrier removal, and can demonstrate the capabilities of aphasic people. There is a danger of confusing aphasic people's experiential expertise about aphasia with knowledge and skills required for a particular job. It is most important that aphasic people are properly trained and equipped, and that attention is paid to any special requirements due to their aphasia. Careful and sympathetic ongoing supervision will be necessary to provide support and to cope with any difficulties that may arise. Only then can aphasic people be expected to feel comfortable in their work and to be empowered by it.

Living with aphasia in residential care

The disability movement in Britain opposes residential care on the grounds that it leads to residents being deprived of decision-making power (e.g. Barnes, 1991, Chapter 6; Finkelstein, 1993; French, 1994c). Townsend's analysis (1981) of institutions for elderly people, based on a number of studies of such institutions in Britain and the USA, concluded that:

> The majority of residents in Homes are placed in a category of enforced dependence. The routine of residential Homes, made

necessary by small staffs and economical administration, and ... an ideology of 'care and attention' rather than the encouragement of self-help and self-management, seems to deprive many residents of the opportunity if not the incentive to occupy themselves and *even to the means of communication*.

(p. 20, emphasis added)

Foster (1991) recognizes that residential care has tended to be seen as a last resort in Britain, and contrasts this with Scandinavian countries where it is viewed more positively. She presents evidence that illustrates the variability of frail elderly people's experience of residential care and argues for changes in standards of provision, for example to afford residents their own defensible space and the facilities to make at least a drink for visitors. Government guidance for residential care homes puts forward principles compatible with social model ideas, emphasizing residents' needs for choice, privacy and dignity. Residential care should offer 'the opportunity to enhance ... [residents'] quality of life and individuals are 'entitled to be involved in all decisions affecting their lives' (DoH/Social Services Inspectorate, 1989, p. 12).

All too little is known about how aphasic people fare in residential settings. Research in the USA suggests that aphasic people 'in institutional environments such as nursing homes have fewer opportunities to communicate than do aphasic people of like age and with similar deficits who live at home' (Holland 1989, p. 2). Clearly, institutional carers have considerable power to facilitate or inhibit communication and, more generally, 'client control'.

We discussed speech and language therapy provision for aphasic people in residential care in Chapter 5, and in Chapter 8 described speech and language therapy initiatives to improve the 'communicative environment' in residential settings by offering training and support to staff.

Gravell (1988) states that 'few care staff in homes are offered explanations and information about communication, and therefore do not value its role in personal fulfilment' (p. 111). There is some evidence that this situation is changing. Speech and language therapists have begun to develop training materials (e.g. Stevens *et al.*, 1992). The 3-year project in Sheffield cited in Chapter 5 (p. 82) (Lester 1993, 1994; Lester, Soord and Trewhitt, 1994) enabled experimentation with a number of different approaches to enhance communication opportunities and the development of ideas about the form and content of training. After some initial resistance to training from long-established care staff, interest increased. The key aspect seemed to be the use of a participative, workshop approach. It may be that the introduction of General National Vocational Qualifications (GNVQs) is creating more positive attitudes than reported by Gravell (1988) towards training in residential homes.

In 1994–5 the DoH funded an ADA project to develop and pilot a training package on communication and communication impairment for care workers. The *Communicate* training, accompanied by a 'user friendly' booklet, is designed to take 2 half-days, the first focusing on communication awareness and the second on coping with communication disability. The training is conducted by a network of speech and language therapists specially recruited and trained for this role. In addition to such training initiatives, literature for care staff has increasingly addressed the issue of communication with residents in institutions (e.g. Maxim and Bryan 1993, 1995).

Bryan and Drew's work (1987) in helping care staff to set up 'communication groups' for residents was described in Chapter 8 (p. 141). Care workers' reports suggest that such groups can have a positive impact on residents' quality of life. Among changes observed by care staff in residents were an increase in the amount and range of conversation between staff and residents, greater tolerance by residents of those with speech problems 'realising that they had something worthwhile to say' and 'an increase in self-esteem'. In addition, 'care staff were often pleasantly surprised at the level of communication achieved and became more aware of the residents' abilities' (Bryan and Drew, 1987, p. 7). In other words, the communication groups served to reveal residents' competence that had formerly been masked either by communication disorder or by factors in the residential setting environment.

Leisure

Drummond (1990) defines leisure as 'activity chosen primarily for its own sake after the practical necessities of life have been attended to' (p. 157). For aphasic people, leisure activities may also provide opportunities to work at their language. In what was almost certainly the first paper to discuss the experience of aphasia associations in different countries, Hubert and Degiovani (1993) identify five roles. In this section we discuss three of these, 'the recreational function', 'solidarity' and 'the quasi-therapeutic role' (pp. 290–1).

Hubert and Degiovani suggest that 'the recreational function is undoubtedly the most universal one'. Leisure activities in which aphasic people can participate are an important aspect of the work of organizations like The Stroke Association and ADA. ADA branch activities have included meetings, outings, fund-raising events, and holidays in Britain and abroad. More 'serious' activities organized by ADA branches, such as awareness raising and intensive speech and language therapy courses, no doubt also have their social side! At national level, ADA organizes an annual 1-day conference, which is primarily aphasic people's own event. The 1994 ADA conference, 'Creative Alternatives' set a new pattern for the afternoon session, with workshops in singing, art and drama. These generated a high level of involvement and much enthusiasm. Workshops at the 1995 conference included painting on ceramics, music with handbells and (by popular request) singing.

Joining others with similar difficulties can have a major impact on quality of life for a disabled person. Other opportunities for interaction may have disappeared. For some, a weekly club meeting may be their only outing and their one chance to meet people from outside their own household. Many aphasic people welcome and benefit from a social environment in which they are given time to express themselves, and structured opportunities for interaction in which they can participate successfully. In Chapter 2 we saw that it can be difficult for someone with aphasia to cope with a more fluid social situation, with extraneous noise, cross-talk and rapidly changing topics. There is, however, a difference between a club founded on shared disability, and one based on an interest that members have in common. To be restricted to the former emphasizes the role as a disabled person, rather than as a person who happens to have an impairment. At least some aphasic people do participate in leisure activities shared with non-disabled people. Our observations suggest that clubs or groups specially for aphasic people are enjoyed by most people who attend them, humour being much in evidence.

Some volunteers may have a tendency to wait on members and to give them the answers in a game or quiz, rather than to allow them to try to do things for themselves. The line between 'providing a supportive environment' and being 'overprotective' is a narrow one and a continuing balancing act. Helpers as well as professionals must make decisions all the time as to when to hold back and when to offer help. A high degree of sensitivity is called for and also (as argued in Chapter 7) training for volunteers, to foster awareness of this delicate balance.

Clubs, speech groups and home-visiting schemes can, as shown in Chapter 7, provide opportunities for speech practice and are a valuable boost to confidence. To some extent, however, they reinforce their members' passive role if they are organized for the communication impaired, usually by non-disabled people, according to the latter's perceptions of need. Involving aphasic people in club management through a committee is one frequently adopted solution to this problem, which can work as long as the committee has some real power! What is crucial for all non-aphasic people providing groups or one-to-one sessions is really to listen to and take on board aphasic people's views and wishes.

Perhaps the main advantage of a group, whether it is for speech and language therapy or social activity, is the help and support members can give each other. We discussed this in Chapter 4 as it pertains to group therapy; here we are concerned with a wider range of groups including those with purely social aims. Both competition and co-operation seem important. The same group members may at one time spur each other on with (hopefully) friendly rivalry, and at another work together on a task or project to achieve an agreed end. The group will also serve as a reference group. Members will see that some have worse problems than they do, or at least that there are some things they can manage as well as others in their group. Joining a group is likely to affect someone's perception of him- or herself as a disabled person. Being introduced into a group of people who are defined as having a similar disability to your own will force you to accept your disability in one sense, but this will not necessarily coincide with psychological acceptance of your 'new self'. Getting to know and like others who share your disability, and feeling valued and liked, may well help you to accept and like yourself again. Aphasia is simply a common denominator within the group. An environment where there is shared experience of aphasia may come as something of a relief, enabling people to relax and feel comfortable with themselves and other members. Within a group of aphasic people, individuals might develop new roles, as group joker, facilitator, supporter or saboteur, for example.

It may be that new members identify to some extent with other members of the group whose problems seem similar to their own. This may encourage the conscious or subconscious setting of personal goals that are more realistic than 'total recovery' goals, as well as fostering maximization of skills. A group can provide on-going opportunities for social support once speech and language therapy ends. This is true of self-help groups, run by aphasic members themselves, of volunteer-led groups, and of other options for social and recreational support that may be available in a given locality. Ideally, there should be a choice among these various kinds of group as no one approach will suit everybody.

The combination of leisure and therapeutic activities to achieve therapeutic aims is one that has been tried in a number of countries, including Britain. One example, in Sweden, was a 5-day residential course for aphasic people and their spouses, led jointly by a speech and language therapist, a psychologist and a neurologist. The course was held well away from hospital. The programme included many 'work' components, including talks about the aetiology, treatment possibilities and prognosis of aphasia, linguistic, psychological and neurological examination for each aphasic participant, daily family therapy and regular individual counselling, daily speech and language therapy groups. The leisure component of the course included talks on topics about the area, such as local cultural history and geography, excursions and (on the borderline between work and leisure) relaxation exercises. Groups were set up so that members mixed with participants other than their spouse, to 'prevent overprotection' (Borenstein, 1993, p. 10). In Poland, 'therapeutic tours' are part of a multidisciplinary treatment programme called Social Communication Oriented Treatment, introduced for patients 'frustrated by the inability to communicate effectively to those in his or her own environment (Pachalska, 1993, p. 160). One therapeutic tour comprises a day-long car rally, during which aphasic people use special symbols to communicate relevant information to the drivers, and undertake tasks 'that require communicative and/or motor skills at "control points"'. There are opportunities to stop at famous buildings such as museums and castles *en route*. Overall, a therapeutic tour provides a great many opportunities for communication, both during the day itself and as the focus for preparatory meetings.

Aphasia may mean unexpected enforced leisure for people of working age. In Chapter 7 we mentioned encountering speech club volunteers who were themselves aphasic people and former patients. Aphasic people are also involved in other kinds of voluntary work, such as visiting newly aphasic people in hospital. Aphasic people in such roles need training and support just like any other volunteers. Aphasic volunteers may in addition have specific requirements because of their impairment. As discussed above in relation to employment, it is essential to take into account the details of the task and the aphasic person's abilities, so that the aphasic person is set up to succeed. Like employment, volunteering can provide status and can be an enriching and empowering experience for the aphasic volunteer.

ORGANIZATIONAL POWER AND APHASIC PEOPLE

In this section we are concerned with the location and distribution of power between organizations and their publics. This is a complex issue. Publicity material and mission statements tell us a certain amount about an organization's orientation towards its clientele. Within large organizations, decision-making processes may differ from one part to another. There may be differing norms of procedure at different levels within an organizational hierarchy. What happens in practice depends on how staff interpret and carry out their designated roles, and will be affected by the personalities and interpersonal skills of individual postholders. Whilst the reader should be aware of such issues, it is beyond the scope of this book to explore them in any detail. We confine ourselves to discussion of three broad rationales for the organization's relationship with aphasic people. Particular organizations may include elements of different models. As we suggested in Chapter 8, there may well be leeway for a professional group, a particular team of workers or an individual employee to adopt an approach other than that dominant in their wider organization.

Professional paternalism

This is sometimes called the medical model. It is closely aligned with, though analytically distinct from, the individual pathology model of disability. As we saw in Chapter 1, the latter is sometimes also called a medical model of disability. The basic tenets of professional paternalism are that specialist knowledge and qualifications mean that professionals know best what is good for their clients, and that professionals' culture and service ethic ensures that they will behave benevolently.

One of the usual implications of being a patient in hospital is that, at least in the short term, all aspects of your life are under the control of doctors, nurses and other health service workers. Even outside hospital, 'patients' lose a certain amount of control over their lives to 'experts' who (they assume or at least hope) have the knowledge to improve their health or reduce their disability. The label 'patient' implies passivity. The suspension of usual responsibilities that is part of the 'sick role' (Parsons, 1951) may be a necessity or at least a welcome relief for the person who is ill. Many people may be only too happy to delegate decision-making power to health professionals whom they trust to act in their best interests.

Someone with continuing disabilities, however, may find it difficult to cast off the role of patient whilst still needing the professionals' services. Aphasia brings a particular disadvantage, in that the ability to express one's requirements, difficulties, wishes, questions, likes, dislikes and opinions is impaired. The person may be given no say in transport arrangements and times for appointments, or may find that health workers, officials and friends speak to their carer rather than directly to them in relation to matters affecting their health, benefits, welfare or activities.

Some voluntary provision is based on the medical model. For example, aphasic people play no part in decision-making structures and processes in relation to The Stroke Association Dysphasic Support in England and Wales and similar services provided (by other voluntary organizations) as the Volunteer Stroke Service in Scotland and as Volunteer Stroke Schemes in Northern Ireland and the Republic of Ireland. Aphasic people's roles are as consumers of services, and there is no doubt that many recipients are quite satisfied both with this role and with the service itself. In some instances an organization's literature uses the designation 'patients' for them. The name of the British voluntary organization Action for Dysphasic Adults also implies paternalism.

Partnership

As stated above, an underlying assumption of the medical model is that 'the professionals know best'. It is increasingly argued that this stance

is inappropriate, and that service providers need to take full account
of disabled people's own perceptions and preferences (e.g. Wood,
1988; Begum and Fletcher, 1995). Beardshaw discusses the possibility of
moving from 'prescriptive" to 'problem-solving' approaches, and concludes
that:

> 'partnership' models of working challenge deep-seated professional
> attitudes and practices, and the power relationships on which they are
> based ... Without a major change in the balance of power from
> professional to client it is hard to see 'partnership' approaches achiev-
> ing anything more than rhetorical success.
>
> *(1988, 44)*

Many speech and language therapists, as we have indicated, genuinely
believe in the idea of a working partnership with service users. The expectation of the CSLT (1991) is that: 'All episodes of care will be negotiated
and agreed between the client/carer and the speech and language
therapist' (p. 21). We are not in a position to judge to what extent the
partnership model is put into practice. Speech and language therapists
work mainly in the NHS where they inevitably feel the influence of the
medical model. Aphasia therapy's uneasy relationship to that model (discussed in Chapter 8) perhaps accounts for some of the tensions that
may arise between speech and language therapists and the medical
profession. Some speech and language therapists may resolve such
tensions by adopting a prescriptive approach, or by failing to explain to
clients and relatives that they are not certain whether a technique will
work. The concept of 'expertise' is central to that of a 'profession'. Speech
and language therapists' expertise constitutes a range of techniques and a
grasp of their likely applicability. We should not underestimate the difficulty for therapists:

- engendered by uncertainty over whether and precisely how they can best
  help particular aphasic clients;
- in counteracting clients' expectations that the therapist will quickly
  discover what 'treatment' is best for them, without thereby losing clients'
  confidence.

Partnership involves a sharing of information with users that is not a
necessary part of the medical model. The role of individual practitioners
here is complemented by that of voluntary organizations. Particularly
relevant in the present context is the information and advice service
provided by ADA, which is described in Chapter 5. The provision of
information to aphasic people, their families and the public also feature
strongly in the aims and activities of aphasia organizations in other
countries (Jordan, 1995b).

The partnership model is seen to some extent in schemes involving volunteers. The aphasic person may be encouraged to identify his or her own priority areas for work, as, for example, in the Stroke Association Dysphasic Support, and in some education-based schemes.

Partnership is also increasing in other ways in voluntary organizations concerned with aphasia. Hubert and Degiovani (1993) detect a trend for aphasia associations in different countries from initial dominance by therapists 'in the creation of the association and the implementation of the administrative structure' towards a sharing of responsibilities with aphasic people, their families and volunteers (p. 294). ADA is a case in point; its decision in the late 1980s to establish local branches can be seen in part as a logical extension of its information and advice service, since many requests could be handled much more effectively locally, and relatives' needs for ongoing support have become increasingly apparent. The development of local branches also offered the opportunity for a shift in emphasis for ADA. ADA considers that continuing speech and language therapy support is important to its branches' success. However, at the local level, much of the 'action' of ADA's title is intended to be not only *for* dysphasic adults, but also *by* such people and their families. At national level, the number of aphasic people on ADA's council (its management body) has increased to three out of 12, with another two places being taken by carers. A representative from each branch and (independent) self-help group form ADA's regional committee, which makes recommendations to council. Aphasic people also play a key role in less formal ways: as volunteers, counsellors, through participation in meetings and conferences, by representing ADA, as speakers and as informal advisers. Overall, aphasic people play a key role in ADA.

As suggested above, the move from the medical model towards partnership approaches is by no means confined to Britain. The Aphasia Association in Ghent, Belgium began in 1980 with little involvement of aphasic people themselves. By 1989 the Association's president could state that:

> Now the patients, their families and the professionals work together constantly ... one of the aims must be the actual participation of the aphasics in the organisation ... We are convinced that, if aphasics are given sufficient responsibility, our form of co-operation will be meaningful and provide enrichment for both parties.
>
> (*Solome, 1989, p. 12*)

Other countries whose aphasia organizations currently belong to this model are the USA and Italy. The Swiss aphasia organization has been predominantly for professionals, but in 1995 was taking the first steps towards greater involvement of aphasic people. One major project in which French-speaking aphasic people from a number of countries have been involved is the film 'Les Mots Perdus' ('Lost Words'), in which aphasic actors portray the lives of four fictional aphasic people in four cities – Quebec, Paris, Geneva and Brussels. Aphasic people have been involved in writing the stories for the film during scriptwriting workshops and, since its launch in 1993, the film has provided a focus for publicity and dissemination of information about aphasia.

Self-determination

We use the term **self-determination** to indicate the degree of initiative taken by aphasic people. Self-determination implies that it is disabled people who set the terms and make the key decisions, as called for by proponents of the social model of disability (Chapter 1, Figure 1.3). Partnership does not preclude self-determination and may contain strong elements of it, but is a 'top-down' approach. Self-determination is a form of self-help in which control rests with aphasic people as individuals or collectively.[2] Professionals may well have an important role in relation to self-determination, for example in providing information or facilities.

One project based on the philosophy of individual self-determination is a day centre run by the local branch of the charity Headway for people aged (normally) between 15 and 64 who have acquired non-progressive brain damage. Whilst its primary clientele are head-injured people, it caters also for some people who have had strokes. It offers a complementary service to those of the NHS speech and language therapy and rehabilitation centre services and can markedly extend the period of rehabilitative input. The two paid half-time staff are supported by a team of volunteers.

The project operates so as to maximize its attenders' control over their own lives. Attenders themselves decide whether and when to attend. This is often the first decision someone has had to make since becoming disabled. Attendance for more than 2 days a week is discouraged, however, since the centre might then be an escape, and its aim is to encourage and enable people to live full and independent lives.

Attenders come from a 30 mile radius, and are responsible for getting themselves to the centre. Some use 'dial-a-ride' or volunteer driver schemes, whilst others are brought by relatives. There is no selection of attenders within the broad criteria described above, and no discharge. Some attenders move on of their own accord, or reduce the time spent there. The centre offers opportunities both for individual activities, including computer-based work, woodwork and pottery, and for group activities such as play readings, an art group, visits and discussions. Attenders can choose to join in a group activity, or to continue working on their own, the only necessarily communal activity being a midday meal. This relaxed, informal approach is possible partly because the centre has its own accommodation, which includes several small rooms.

The Headway centre aims to find out what each attender wants to do and can do, facilitated by the helpers. Every new attender discusses with a member of staff what activities will help him or her, and this discussion forms the basis for an agreed programme tailored to suit the attender's own interest, experience and perceived rehabilitation needs. There is thus a considerable focus on self-motivation.

Hubert and Degiovani (1993) suggest that many aphasic people capable of taking on the responsibilities of managing an aphasia organization 'tend to avoid the association for fear of being categorized as *disabled* (p. 294, italics in the original). There are, however, many examples of aphasic people themselves controlling their organizations.

In Britain, ADA sponsors a growing number of self-help groups. These are run entirely by aphasic people, who can use a speech and language therapist as a resource. Commenting on her experience of one such group, Margot said:

> My first meeting with the self help group ... was ... I didn't want to be part of it ... I was looking for people who were ... my colleague types, who were able to communicate and outward-going. But it's changed my life, meeting people at the self-help groups, because they were very bright, many of them very very bright, successful people before their strokes and they're re-adapting again as I am, to a totally new life, and being very positive. ... The self help group helped me a lot. ... I've made lots and lots of friends, from the self help group, going on trips and seeing parts of London that we wouldn't have had time for whilst we were working. ... There are bonuses.
>
> (*ADA Personal Insights audiocassette, 1995*)

The self-help groups include activities to help others, as well as themselves. One group persuaded the authorities to install a pelican crossing on the busy road outside their local hospital. Another met with consultants employed by British Telecommunications to consider services offered to disabled people.

Collective self-determination is more highly developed elsewhere in Europe, where aphasic people run their own organizations such as 'Se Comprendre' (in Brussels), the Belgian Federation of French-speaking Aphasics, the Association of Aphasics in Norway and the National Federation of French Aphasics. There are many self-help groups in Germany organized by aphasic people themselves. Outside Europe, countries with organizations of aphasic people include Frenchspeaking Canada (Le Dorze, Croteau and Joanette, 1993) and Japan. The number of Japanese Aphasia Peer Circles has increased rapidly in recent years (Sasanuma, 1993) to 130 by early 1995. The AIA, itself run by a Board of Directors comprising aphasic and formerly aphasic people, holds its general assembly in a different country each year. Its international congresses in 1989 and 1993 included a number of papers given by aphasic people. In 1994 AIA published an *International Guide for Aphasics*, which lists relevant organizations in 32 countries.

The self-determination model is beginning to filter into speech and language therapy practice in Britain. This is due partly to the assertiveness of a few aphasic individuals who have challenged the traditional assumptions about professional/client roles, and forged new relationships in which they (aphasic clients) set the agenda. No less important has been the responsiveness of their therapists, their openness to new ideas and their willingness to change established ways of working. There is a growing awareness among speech and language therapists of the disability movement and considerable interest in promoting equal opportunities for communication-impaired people (Parr, Pound and Marshall, 1995; Trewhitt, 1995). This is evidenced by the focus on such issues by therapists, with the help of aphasic people, at a number of events from 1993 on. These include the British Aphasiology Society (BAS) conferences in 1993 and 1995, study days organized jointly by the BAS and ADA on 'Power and Empowerment', and ADA's 'Self Help Workshops', which provide a forum where therapists and aphasic people wishing to set up self-help groups can work through the issues together. A research project at London's City University to explore the effects of aphasia on everyday life and to develop life-enhancing strategies has involved aphasic people both as researchers and as an advisory group (Parr and Gilpin, 1995).

Evidence of social model thinking and practice also emerges from papers about aphasia therapy in other countries. A clear example is given by Le Dorze, Croteau and Joanette (1993) in French-speaking Canada. They base their discussion on the WHO categorization of impairment, disability and handicap (explained in Chapter 1), nevertheless explicitly distinguishing between aphasia being interpreted as 'a significant handicap which prevents the aphasic person from functioning normally in society' and aphasia 'as society's inability to integrate individuals who function differently from most others' (p. 97). This leads to an approach to intervention that 'includes relatives, friends and colleagues of aphasic individuals, in the sense that compensatory mechanisms leading to more effective communication between aphasic and nonaphasic persons could be identified and implemented to decrease aphasia's handicap'. 'Public advocacy' is suggested as an additional mode of intervention, since: 'Better understanding of aphasia could lead to better recognition and fulfilment of aphasic persons' needs.'

APHASIA AND SOCIETY

The low level of understanding about aphasia in our society has far-reaching implications. It means that most people have little knowledge about how best to communicate with an aphasic person. It accounts, to some extent, for the relatively poor development of aphasia services in some health authorities. As the CST Aphasia Working Party (1989) made clear, responsibility here rests not only with 'medical and general management' but also with 'speech therapy management itself' (p. 7). Furthermore, it results in national policy being based on inadequate information. The most recent government survey of disabled adults in Britain carried out by the Office of Population Censuses and Surveys (OPCS) (Martin, Meltzer and Elliot, 1988) provides an example. Rossiter (1989) shows that OPCS handling of communication disabilities has conceptual and practical limitations that almost certainly led to underestimation of both the numbers of communication-impaired people and the severity of communication disabilities.

Swelling the numbers of people who are aware of aphasia and have a basic understanding of it is an important first step towards empowerment of aphasic people. As we saw in Chapter 2, the frustrations stemming from the impairment itself can be compounded by other people's adverse reactions and behaviour. Lack of awareness can lead also to unintentional discrimination against aphasic people. One project we encountered initially classed quite severely aphasic people without significant mobility difficulties as 'unimpaired' and therefore as not requiring any services on leaving hospital. This happened because the dominant medical stereotype of disability, which 'sees' only visible, physical impairments, had been a major influence on the project's criteria and procedures.

The profile of aphasia needs to be raised in a number of arenas. Central government has the power to ensure that policies do not disadvantage communication-impaired people. Health commissioners play a key role in allocating NHS resources so have the power to improve funding for aphasia services. Various providers of health and social care need to be aware of aphasia, and the fact that it can be treated, to encourage referral, to ease their interactions with aphasic people and to foster good working relationships among different professions. Colleges may provide educational opportunities for aphasic people. The words 'aphasia' and 'dysphasia' need to be promoted so that they become common currency, though having two terms in Britain is bound to be confusing. Hubert and Degiovani (1993) identify 'publicising aphasia' as a role of aphasia associations. Public awareness of aphasia would reduce misunderstandings and obviate the need for continual explanations. It could also have indirect effects, for example in relation to resources and professional interest. The key information in all publicity should be the underlying competence of aphasic people as this is an essential prerequi-site to changing attitudes.

We must recognize that, as a cause, aphasia may not be of immediate appeal to the mass media. The response to ADA's occasional radio fund-raising slots – in terms of correspondence as well as donations – suggests, however, that it does strike a chord with many people. Our impression is that media coverage of aphasia in Britain and elsewhere has increased in recent years, probably because of a number of factors, including:

- greater awareness and media concern with disability issues more generally;
- events like the British Telecommunications' sponsored 'Speech Watch' (formerly 'Speak Week');
- attention gained by the work of voluntary organizations and individual speech and language therapists;
- media interest in famous people who have become aphasic.

Pachalska (1993) discusses some similar factors in Poland. Communication is so taken for granted that it is difficult to convey what its sudden loss is like. Aphasia organizations in many countries are attempting to do just this with, for example, some imaginative publicity material, training videos, a film (see pp. 177–8) and, whenever possible, radio and television interviews. Portrayal of aphasia in the mainstream arts has been scant, one exception being a play first produced in the late 1980s, 'The Traveller', which centres around the principal character's aphasia (see Appendix B).

Making an impact may be easier at a local level than nationally. Groups such as ADA branches and Stroke Association Dysphasic Support services fundraise through social events that may make the local news. Activities that take aphasic people into the community such as individual or group outings may provide opportunities for 'equal status contact' (Block and Yuker, 1979) but probably only if a facilitator is available.

The ADA *Communicate* training, discussed above in relation to residential care, also has considerable potential both to raise awareness and to begin development of the necessary communication skills among all those whose lives bring them into contact with aphasic and other communication-impaired people. *Communicate* is being taken up by NHS trusts, Social Services departments and consortia of residential care homes for a far wider range of staff than initially anticipated. Its application has been recognized for such groups as nurses, occupational therapists, day care workers, home helps and home care workers, GP receptionists, clerical, domestic, maintenance and portering staff in care settings, ambulance service staff and informal carers. A modified version of *Communicate* for the commercial and retail sector is planned.

The final role attributed to aphasia associations by Hubert and Degiovani (1993) is as 'defense of the rights of persons with aphasia and their families'. Publicity can be an unanticipated outcome of a request for help in this regard, as illustrated by a recent court case in which the speech and language therapist and ADA took an advocacy role. The case concerned a person who became aphasic, with very limited speech, as the result of an assault. A policeman visited him six times to take his statement. This was accepted by the magistrates court only after ADA supplied literature about aphasia that reassured the court that an aphasic person could be a reliable witness, and the defendant was remanded in custody. At the trial in the Crown Court a video camera was trained on the witness stand and monitors were provided for the judge, barristers, defendant and jury, so that the aphasic person could use his communication notebook, plans and photographs to give some of his evidence by writing, drawing and pointing. He also used gesture and gave yes/no answers. With the agreement of the judge and barristers, the phrases 'say that again' and 'I can't find the words' were written on paper for the aphasic witness's use. To avoid tiring the witness, frequent short adjournments of the court were agreed. These arrangements were unprecedented (RCSLT Bulletin, 1995a). The case received coverage in the three main national broadsheet newspapers.

Awareness and knowledge about aphasia are not, by themselves, enough to create more communication opportunities for aphasic people. Skills in using simple communication strategies are also required. An interviewer on a radio programme for (and presented by) disabled people spoke rapidly in convoluted sentences and 'lost' the highly intelligent, articulate aphasic person being interviewed. The interviewee's competence was, in effect, masked. Before the criminal court case cited above, the prosecuting barrister visited the aphasic witness and took advice from his speech and language therapist 'on his comprehension level and how best to obtain his evidence' (RCSLT Bulletin, 1995a, p. 1). In addition, the speech and language therapist was permitted to provide both barristers with advice in court. The defendant was convicted. The prosecution team described the aphasic person as 'an excellent witness'.

Facilitated communication, with a speech and language therapist or other trained person acting as interpreter, is undoubtedly needed in the absence of widespread training of those in contact with aphasic people. This could prove expensive in speech and language therapists' time and difficult to justify except in special circumstances. Consideration could be given to the deployment of appropriately trained speech and language therapy assistants or even volunteers. It needs emphasizing that success would depend on the training and supervision provided by speech and language therapists. There is a strong case for a demonstration project to develop training along the lines pioneered by the Aphasia Centre – North

York and to pilot such a scheme in Britain. Families and friends of aphasic people, health and welfare workers and volunteers working with aphasic people are the priority groups for communication strategy training, but ideally it should be more generally available.

Arato and Kagan (1995; also Kagan, 1995) provide a dramatic demonstration of the impact of training for conversation partners in samples on video of two meetings between an aphasic person and a young neurologist. The doctor is gentle and sympathetic, but is almost totally unable to elicit information from the aphasic person, who presents as dull and diffident. The doctor's feelings about this interaction and image of the aphasic person would undoubtedly have been negative. In addition to the evident discomfort for the conversation partners at the time, these impressions might conceivably have affected the doctor's subsequent use of his power to make treatment decisions to the disadvantage of the aphasic person. A fortnight later, after the doctor has received some training, a second conversation between the same two conversation partners shows marked contrasts. The doctor 'follows a similar line of questioning but slightly alters his rate of speech, and immediately starts making extensive use of pen and paper to write key words and verify ... responses' (Kagan, 1995, p. 16). (The pen and writing pad were available but unused during the first interview.) Both partners are more relaxed; the aphasic person now appears intelligent, animated and friendly; the doctor is much happier; and successful exchange of information transpires. Most people would assume that there had been a significant improvement in the aphasic person's communicative ability, but in fact he 'received no specific treatment in the two weeks between the videos' (ibid.) Without the training received by the doctor, the real person would have remained hidden behind the mask of aphasia.

This example shows how an aphasic person's competence can be revealed. Our assertion is that revealing this competence on a wide scale is crucial to removal of the barriers that limit aphasic people's control over their own lives, in other words, for empowerment. It remains to summarize the action required for this to happen.

Political action is required because aphasic people's life chances are determined to some extent by the position of disabled people in society. The acceptance of disability as a human rights issue and the corollary of comprehensive anti-discrimination legislation are necessary to provide a framework for equality. As we explained in Chapter 6 (p. 105), comprehensive anti-discrimination legislation has been introduced in some countries but not, despite many attempts, in Britain (RADAR, 1994; *Disability Now*, 1995). This top-down approach is both advocated and complemented by the grass roots political action of the disability movement. The movement understandably – perhaps inevitably –

underplays the differing implications of different impairments, and since communication is its principal weapon it is not surprising that people with communication impairments tend to be underrepresented. There is a need for the disability movement to incorporate what is required to empower people with communication impairments into its ideas and activities.

In Chapter 8 we have looked in some detail at the professional action required of speech and language therapists. Adoption of the social model of disability should produce a new strength of purpose in the profession and give aphasia therapists a wider perspective that could prove invaluable in the jostle for the resources needed for aphasia services within health care quasi-markets. Seeing themselves and their expertise and skills as a resource for aphasic people should be an enlightening and empowering experience for aphasia therapists. This is not to say that it will be easy. The individual pathology model of disability is, if possible, even more deeply ingrained in health care than elsewhere in society. There will be conflicts at times and therapists will undoubtedly find themselves slipping back into old ways of thinking and working.

Action required in the wider community includes the work of national and local voluntary organizations. Some reorientation of programmes will be necessary if they are to take on board the implications of the social model of disability. They should be able to look to the disability movement and the speech and language therapy profession for support in this. Volunteers should insist on training in strategies to reveal competence. They can do a great deal by talking about aphasia to others in their social networks. Aphasic people's friends and relatives must be prepared to acknowledge their own needs and recognize that these may at times conflict with those of 'their' aphasic person.

Aphasic people testify to the value of managing and belonging to their own organizations, and by working together they demonstrate their competence. They also need to be conscious that their aphasia is not solely their problem. With the help of facilitators and advocates, some of whom may also be aphasic, they can take their rightful share of power. They are, ultimately, their own best ambassadors, and the real experts on aphasia. The challenge for the non-aphasic community is to listen to aphasic people and act with them according to their perspectives. Only this will enable policies and practices in relation to aphasic people that foster their empowerment.

Endnotes
[1]This is not to say that rehabilitation workers do not already act in all these ways at least to some extent. The change called for is in their overview of their role.

[2]This may appear to be stating the obvious, but the label 'self-help' can be deceptive. It may be applied, for example, to distinguish a volunteer-run group from a therapist-controlled group. The test in every case must be: 'who holds decision-making power?'

References

Note: n.d. = no date.

Action for Dysphasic Adults (1982) *ADA Newsletter*, No. 4, 12–13.

Action for Dysphasic Adults (1990) *Stroke and Dysphasia: Drawing the Picture Together*, ADA, London.

Action for Dysphasic Adults (1995) *National Directory: National Register of Language Opportunities for those with Dysphasia and their Families*, ADA, London, volumes 2–4.

Age Concern London (1995) *Home Comforts: Home Support for Disabled Older People*, Age Concern London, London.

Anderson, R. (1988) The consequences of stroke for the family. In King's Fund Forum, *The Treatment of Stroke: Programme and Abstracts*, King's Fund, London.

Anderson, R. (1992) *The Aftermath of Stroke,* Cambridge University Press, Cambridge.

Aphasia Centre – North York (1994a) History (Information sheet). Aphasia Centre, Ontario.

Aphasia Centre – North York (1994b) Note to families and friends of our aphasic members (Information sheet), Aphasia Centre, Ontario.

Aphasia Centre – North York (1994c) Volunteer opportunities at the Aphasia Centre (Information sheet), Aphasia Centre, Ontario.

Arato, P. and Kagan, A. (1995) The North York Aphasia Centre Ontario: the work and the people, Action for Dysphasic Adults eleventh annual Mary Law memorial lecture, 5 June 1995, London.

Association of County Councils/Association of Metropolitan Authorities (1995) *Who Gets Community Care?* Association of Metropolitan Authorities, London.

Association Internationale Aphasie (ed.) (1994) *International Guide for Aphasics*, AIA, Brussels.

Baldock, J. and Ungerson, C. (1994) *Becoming Consumers of Community Care,*

Joseph Rowntree Foundation, York.

Barnes, C. (1991) *Disabled People in Britain and Discrimination*, Hurst/British Council of Organizations of Disabled People, London.

Barnett, E. (1994) Using outcome measures to improve the service, *College of Speech and Language Therapists Bulletin*, **507** (July), 12–14.

Basso, A. (1993) Therapy for aphasia in Italy, in *Aphasia Treatment: World Perspectives* (eds A.L. Holland and M.M. Forbes), Chapman & Hall, London, pp. 1–23.

Beardshaw, V. (1988) *Last on the List: Community Services for People with Physical Disabilities*, King's Fund Institute, London.

Begum, N. and Fletcher, S. (1995) *Improving Disability Services: The way forward for health and social services,* Living Options Partnership Paper no. 3, King's Fund, London.

Block, J.R. and Yuker, H.E. (1979) Attitudes towards disability are the key, *Rehabilitation Digest*, **10**, 2–3.

Borden, W.A. (1962) Psychological aspects of stroke: patient and family, *Annals of Internal Medicine*, **57** (4), 689–92.

Borenstein, P. (1993) *Depression and Aphasia*, The Mary Law lecture, 20 April, ADA, London.

Brindley, P., Copeland, M., Demain, C. and Martyn, P. (1989) A comparison of the speech of ten chronic Broca's aphasics following intensive and non-intensive speech therapy, *Aphasiology*, **3** (8), 695–707.

British Aphasiology Society (1993) *Purchasing Speech and Language Therapy Services for People with Aphasia*, British Aphasiology Society, London.

Brooks, N., McKinlay, W., Symington, C. *et al.* (1987) Return to work within the first seven years of severe head injury, *Brain Injury*, **1** (1), 5–19.

Brumfitt, S. and Clarke, P. (1983) An application of psychotherapeutic techniques to the management of aphasia, in *Aphasia Therapy*, (eds C. Code and D. Muller), Edward Arnold, London, pp. 88–100.

Bryan, K. and Drew, S. (1987) The benefits of therapy for elderly people in care, *Speech Therapy in Practice,* **3** (2), 6–9.

Bryan, K.L. and Drew, S. (1989) A survey of communication disability in an elderly population in residential care. *International Journal of Rehabilitation Research*, **12** (3), 330–3.

Bury, M. (1991) The sociology of chronic illness: a review of research and prospects, *Sociology of Health and Illness*, **13** (4), 452–68.

Byng, S. (1989) Aphasia European Congress. *British Aphasiology Society Newsletter*, July, 3–4.

Byng, S. (1990) Should we be more creative with our volunteers? *Speech Therapy in Practice*, **6** (6), 14–15.

Byng, S. and Jones, E. (1993) Interactional coding of aphasia therapy. Presentation at British Aphasiology Society Conference, Warwick University.

Bynoe, I., Oliver, M. and Barnes, C. (1991) *Equal Rights for Disabled People: The case for a new law*, Institute for Public Policy Research, London.

Camp, L. (n.d.) Our Monday group. *New Horizons*, Radwinter Hospital Adult Education Group, **2**, 8–10.

Campling, J. (ed) (1981) *Images of Ourselves*, Routledge and Kegan Paul, London.

City Dysphasic Group (1989) *In Our Own Words – Dysphasic People Talking*, Action for Dysphasic Adults, London.

Cohen, N.V. (1987) Notepads for people with impaired speech. *College of Speech Therapists Bulletin*, **425** (Sept.), 30.

College of Speech and Language Therapists (CSLT) (1991) *Communicating Quality: Professional Standards for Speech and Language Therapists*, College of Speech and Language Therapists, London.

College of Speech and Language Therapists Bulletin (1993) College responds to Tomlinson report, **489** (January), 1.

College of Speech Therapists (CST) Aphasia Working Party (1989) Good practice in aphasia therapy. *College of Speech Therapists Bulletin*, **449** (Sept.), 7–10.

Coltheart, M., Sartori, G. and Job, R. (1987) *Cognitive Neuropsychology of Language*. Lawrence Erlbaum Associates, London.

Coughlan, A.K. and Humphrey, M. (1982) Presenile stroke: Long term outcome for patients and their families. *Rheumatology and Rehabilitation*, **21**, 115–22.

Cutler, T. and Waine, B. (1994) *Managing the Welfare State*, Berg, Oxford.

Dalley, G. (1988) *Ideologies of Caring*. Macmillan, London.

David, R.M., Enderby, P. and Bainton, D. (1982) Treatment of acquired aphasia: speech therapists and volunteers compared. *Journal of Neurology, Neurosurgery and Psychiatry*, **45**, 957–61.

David, R.M., Enderby, P. and Bainton, D. (1983) Response to T R Pring 1, *British Journal of Disorders of Communication*, **18**, 73–7.

Davies, P. and van der Gaag, A. (1993) A sound investment? *College of Speech and Language Therapists Bulletin*, **494** (June), 4–6.

Davis, G.A. and Wilcox, M.J. (1981) Incorporating parameters of natural conversation in aphasia treatment, in *Language Intervention Strategies in Adult Aphasia*, (ed. R.Chapey), Williams and Wilkins, Baltimore.

Department of Education and Science (1972) *Speech Therapy Services*, Report of the Committee appointed by the Secretaries of State for Education and Science, for the Social Services, for Scotland and Wales in July 1969. (Quirk Report), HMSO, London.

Department of Health (1989a) *Caring for people: Community Care in the Next Decade and Beyond*, CM. 849, HMSO, London.

Department of Health (1989b) *Working for Patients*, CM. 555, HMSO, London.

Department of Health/Social Services Inspectorate (1989) *Homes Are For Living In*, HMSO, London.

Department of Health (1991, 1995) *The Patient's Charter*, HMSO, London.

Department of Health (1992) *The Health of the Nation: a Strategy for Health in England*, HMSO, London.

Department of Health (1995) *NHS Responsibilities for Meeting Continuing Health Care Needs*, HSG (95) 8/LAC (95) 5, DoH, London.

Disability Alliance (1995) *Disability Rights Handbook*, 20th Edition April

1995–April 1996, Disability Alliance Educational and Research Association, London.

Disability Now (1995) What's on offer, February, p. 2.

Dodd, M., McAuslan, S., Smith, B. and Archer, B. (1992) Do people with aphasia return to work? *College of Speech and Language Therapists Bulletin*, 485, September, p. 8.

Drummond, A. (1990) Leisure activity after stroke. *International Disability Studies*, **12**, 157–60.

Duggan, M. (1995) *Primary Health Care: A Prognosis*, Institute for Public Policy Research, London.

Eastwood, J. and Thompson, P. (1995) The generic health care worker: the idea that won't lie down and die. *College of Speech and Language Therapists Bulletin*, **517** (May), 10–11.

Edelman, G. and Greenwood, R. (eds) (1992) *Jumbly Words, and Rights Where Wrongs Should Be: The Experience of Aphasia from the Inside*, Far Communications, Kibworth.

Ellis, A.W. and Young, A.W. (1988) *Human Cognitive Neuropsychology*, Lawrence Erlbaum Associates, London.

Ellis, K. (1993) *Squaring the Circle: User and Carer Participation in Needs Assessment*, Joseph Rowntree Foundation, London.

Enderby, P. (1992) Outcome measures in speech therapy: impairment, disability, handicap and distress. *Health Trends*, **24** (2), 61–4.

Enderby, P. and Davies, P. (1989) Communication disorders: planning a service to meet the needs. *British Journal of Disorders of Communication*, **24**, 301–32.

Fielden, N. (1994) Measuring and monitoring efficiency of treatment, *College of Speech and Language Therapists Bulletin*, **505** (May), 9–10.

Finkelstein, V. (1991) Disability: an administrative challenge (the health and welfare heritage), in *Social Work, Disabled People and Disabling Environments* (ed. M. Oliver), Jessica Kingsley, London, pp. 19–39.

Finkelstein, V. (1993) Disability: a social challenge or an administrative responsibility? in *Disabling Barriers – Enabling Environments* (eds J. Swain, V. Finkelstein, S. French and M. Oliver), Sage, London, pp. 34–43.

Finkelstein, V. and French, S. (1993) Towards a psychology of disability, in *Disabling Barriers – Enabling Environments* (eds J. Swain, V. Finkelstein, S. French, and M. Oliver), Sage, London, pp. 26–33.

Flowers, J. and Korczak, J. (1981) Coping with a stroke in the family: a project in Hertfordshire to help stroke patients and their families at home. *Social Work Service*, **26**, 40–5.

Floyd, M. (1991) Overcoming barriers to employment, in *Disability and Social Policy* (ed. G. Dalley), Policy Studies Institute, London, pp. 210–35.

Foggitt, E. (1987) Give our skills the respect they deserve. *Speech Therapy in Practice*, **2** (4), 29.

Foster, P. (1991) Residential care for frail elderly people: a positive reassessment, *Social Policy and Administration*, **25** (2) June, 108–20.

French, S. (1993a) Disability, impairment or something in between? in *Disabling*

Barriers – Enabling Environments (eds J. Swain, V. Finkelstein, S. French, and M. Oliver), Sage, London, pp. 17–25.

French, S. (1993b) What's so great about independence? in *Disabling Barriers – Enabling Environments* (eds J. Swain, F. Finklestein, S. French and M. Oliver), Sage, London, p. 44–48.

French, S. (1994a) The disabled role. Chapter 4 in *On Equal Terms: Working with Disabled People* (ed. S. French), Butterworth-Heinemann, Oxford, pp. 47–60.

French, S. (1994b) Disabled people and professional practice. Chapter 8 in *On Equal Terms: Working with Disabled People* (ed. S. French), Butterworth-Heinemann, Oxford, pp. 103–18.

French, S. (1994c) Institutional and community living. Chapter 9 in *On Equal Terms: Working with Disabled People* (ed. S. French), Butterworth-Heinemann, Oxford, pp. 119–35.

Geddes, J., Poulter, J. and Chamberlain, Prof A. (1995) Dysphasia support team. *College of Speech and Language Therapists Bulletin*, **516** (April), 10–12.

Gibbs, D. (1995) Incapacity Benefit: a contradiction that can't last. *Disability Now*, April, p. 11.

Goddard, E. (1994) *Voluntary Work: A study carried out on behalf of the Home Office as part of the 1992 General Household Survey*, HMSO, London.

Goffman, E. (1968) *Stigma: Notes on the Management of Spoiled Identity*, Penguin, Harmondsworth.

Goodglass, H. and Kaplan, E. (1983) *The Assessment of Aphasia and Related Disorders*, 2nd edn, Lea and Febiger, Philadelphia.

Gravell, R. (1988) *Communication Problems in Elderly People*, Croom Helm, London and Sydney.

Green, G. (1984) Communication in aphasia therapy: some of the procedures and issues involved. *British Journal of Disorders of Communication*, **19**, 35–40.

Griffith, V.E. (1975) Volunteer scheme for dysphasic and allied problems in stroke patients. *British Medical Journal*, 5984, 633–5.

Griffith, V.E. (1980) Observations on patients dysphasic after stroke. *British Medical Journal*, **281**, 1608–9.

Griffith, V.E. (n.d.) *Volunteer Stroke Scheme Handbook*. Chest, Heart and Stroke Association, London.

Griffith, V.E. and Miller, C.L. (1980) Volunteer stroke scheme for dysphasic patients with stroke. *British Medical Journal*, **281**, 1605–7.

Griffiths, R. (1988) *Community Care: Agenda for Action*, HMSO, London.

Hammen, V., Yorkston, K. and Beukelman, D. (1989) Pausal and speech duration characteristics as a function of speaking rate in normal and Parkinsonian dysarthric subjects, in *Recent Advances in Clinical Dysarthria* (eds K. Yorkston and D. Buekelman), College Hill, Boston.

Herrmann, M., Johannsen-Horbach, H. and Wallesch, C.-W. (1993) The psychosocial aspects of aphasia, in *Living with aphasia: Psychosocial issues* (eds D. Lafond, R. DeGiovani, Y. Joanette, J. Ponzio and M. Taylor Sarno), Singular Publishing Group, Inc., San Diego, California, pp. 188–205.

Hills, J. (1993) *The Future of Welfare: A guide to the debate*, Joseph Rowntree Foundation, York, p. 8.

Holland, A. (1982) Observing functional communication of aphasic adults. *Journal of Speech and Hearing Disorders*, **47**, 50–6.

Holland, A.L. (1989) Some psychosocial factors in aphasia. 6th Mary Law memorial lecture. Action for Dysphasic Adults, London.

Holland, A.L. (1991) Pragmatic aspects of intervention in aphasia. *Journal of Neurolinguistics*, **6** (2), 197–211.

Holland, A.L. (1993) Preface in *Aphasia Treatment: World Perspectives* (eds A.L. Holland and M.M. Forbes), Chapman & Hall, London.

Hopkins, A. (1975) The need for speech therapy for dysphasia following stroke, *Health Trends*, **7**, 58–60.

Howard, D. (1986) Beyond randomised controlled trials: the case for effective case studies of the effects of treatment in aphasia, *British Journal of Disorders of Communication,* **21** (1), 89–102.

Huber, W., Springer, L. and Willmes, K. (1993) Approaches to aphasia therapy in Aachan. In *Aphasia Treatment: World Perspectives* (eds A.L. Holland and M.M. Forbes), Chapman & Hall, London, pp. 55–86.

Hubert, M.D. and Degiovani, R. (1993) Associations for persons with aphasia. In *Living with Aphasia: Psychosocial Issues* (eds D. Lafond, R. Degiovani, Y. Joanette, J. Ponzio and M. Taylor Sarno), Singular Publishing Group Inc., San Diego, California, pp. 279–301.

Hull, B. and Wilson, G. (1994) Communicating audit: friend or foe. *College of Speech and Language Therapists Bulletin*, **506** (June), 11–12.

Hunter, D.J. (ed.) (1988) *Bridging the Gap: Case management and advocacy for people with physical handicaps*. King Edward's Hospital Fund for London, London.

Hutton, W. (1995) *The State We're In*, Jonathan Cape, London.

Illich, I. (1976) *Medical Nemesis*, Penguin, Harmondsworth.

Ireland, C. and Black, M. (1992) Living with aphasia: the insight story. In *Working Papers in Linguistics*, University College, London, pp. 355–8.

Ireland, C. and Wotton, G. (1993). *Time to talk,* ADA Counselling project, Department of Health Report, Action for Dysphasic Adults, London.

Jones, E. (1986) Building the foundations for sentence production in a non-fluent aphasic. *British Journal of Disorders of Communication*, **21**, 63–82.

Jordan, F.M., Worrall, L.E., Hickson, L.M.H. and Dodd, B.J. (1993) The evaluation of intervention programmes for communicatively impaired elderly people *European Journal of Disorders of Communication*, **28**, 63–85.

Jordan, L. (1989a) Family or volunteer? *Therapy Weekly*, **16** (1) 20 July, 9.

Jordan, L. (1989b) Volunteers: the case for training. *Speech Therapy in Practice*, **5** (3) August, 7–8.

Jordan, L. (1990) Weighing up the cost of volunteers. S*peech Therapy in Practice*, Update, 8 November, v–vi.

Jordan, L. (1991) A profile of aphasia services in three health districts. *British Journal of Disorders of Communication*, **26**, 293–315.

Jordan, L. (1994) NHS changes – the impact on services. *College of Speech and Language Therapists Bulletin*, **504** (April), 9–11.

Jordan, L. (1995a) Clients as claimants: the role of speech and language therapists. *Royal College of Speech and Language Therapists Bulletin*, **521** (September), 8–9.

Jordan, L. (1995b) Organizations concerned with aphasia: an international survey. Conference Paper, British Aphasiology Society International Conference, University of York, September.

Kagan, A. (1995) Revealing the competence of aphasic adults through conversation: a challenge to health professionals. *Topics in Stroke Rehabilitation*, **2**(1), 15–28.

Kagan, A. and Gailey, G. (1993) Functional is not enough: Training of conversation partners for aphasic adults, in *Aphasia Treatment: World Perspectives* (eds A.L. Holland and M.M. Forbes), Chapman & Hall, London, pp. 199–225.

Kaiser, W. and Jordan, L. Pathways of care for aphasic stroke patients, in preparation.

Kay, J., Lesser R. and Coltheart, M. (1992) *Psycholinguistic Assessments of Language Processing in Aphasia*, Lawrence Erlbaum Associates, London.

King's Fund Forum on Stroke (1988) *The Treatment of Stroke: Consensus Statement*, King Edward's Hospital Fund for London, London.

Kinsella, G.J. and Duffy, F.D. (1978) The spouse of the aphasic patient, in *The Management of Aphasia* (eds R. Hoops and Y. Lebrun) Neurolinguistics Volume 8, Swets and Zeitlinger B.V., Amsterdam and Lisse, pp. 26–49.

Kinsella, G.J. and Duffy, F.D. (1979) Psychosocial readjustment in the spouses of stroke patients, *Scandinavian Journal of Rehabilitation Medicine*, **11**, 129–32.

Kinsella, G.J. and Duffy, F.D. (1980) Attitudes towards disability expressed by spouses of stroke patients, *Scandinavian Journal of Rehabilitation Medicine*, 12, 73–6.

Klein, R. (1995) *The New Politics of the NHS*, 3rd edn, Longman, London.

Körner, E. (1983) NHS steering group on health services information, *A report from working group C: Paramedical services*, Department of Health and Social Security, London.

Law, D. and Paterson, B. (1980) *Living After a Stroke*, Souvenir Press, London.

Lebrun, Y. (1978) The inside of aphasia, in *The Management of Aphasia* (eds R. Hoops and Y. Lebrun) Neurolinguistics Volume 8, Swets and Zeitlinger, B.V., Amsterdam and Lisse, pp. 50–5.

Lebrun, Y., Lelwux, C., Fery, C. *et al.* (1978) Aphasia and fitness to drive, in *The Management of Aphasia* (eds R. Hoops and Y. Lebrun) Neurolinguistics volume 8, Swets and Zeitlinger, B.V., Amsterdam and Lisse, pp. 56–65.

Le Dorze, G., Croteau, C. and Joanette, Y. (1993) Perspectives on Aphasia Intervention in French-Speaking Canada, in *Aphasia Treatment: World Perspectives* (eds A.L. Holland and M.M. Forbes), Chapman & Hall, London, pp. 87–114.

Lendrem, W. (1994) Clinical decision analysis and the selection of aphasic patients for active treatment, PhD thesis, Faculty of Medicine, University of Newcastle.

Lendrem, W. and Hurst, L. (1990) Communication disability and handicap in residents living in three residential care homes in Newcastle on Tyne, unpublished report.

Lendrem, W. and Stamp, S. (1985) North Tyneside stroke relative support group, *College of Speech Therapists Bulletin*, October, 10.

Leroy, W. (1992) Volunteer Stroke Service: exhausting but exhilarating, *College of Speech and Language Therapists Bulletin*, 485 (September), 8.

Lesser, R. and Milroy, L. (1993) *Linguistics and Aphasia, Psycholinguistic and Pragmatic Aspects of Intervention*, Longman, London.

Lesser, R. and Watt, M. (1978) Untrained community help in the rehabilitation of stroke sufferers with language disorders, *British Medical Journal*, **2**, 1045–8.

Lester, R. (1993) *Care of the Elderly Project Volunteer Scheme: a report on a trial scheme using volunteers to work with residents with communication disabilities in local authority homes for older people*, Sheffield Communication Therapy, Sheffield.

Lester, R. (1994) Residential care: 'Towards a better understanding', *College of Speech and Language Therapists Bulletin*, **512** (December), 11–12.

Lester, R., Soord, G. and Trewhitt, P. (1994) *Towards a Better Understanding*, Sheffield Communication Therapists/Family and Community Services Training and Development, Sheffield.

Lincoln, N., McGuirk, E., Mulley, G. *et al.* (1984) The effectiveness of Speech Therapy for aphasic stroke patients. A randomised controlled trial. *The Lancet*, **i**, 1197–200.

Logan, K. (1994) From the inside, *Speaking Up*, Issue 31 (Winter), 6–7.

Lomas, J., Pickard, L., and Mohide, A. (1987) Patient versus clinician item generation for quality of life measures. The case of language disabled adults, *Medical Care*, **25**(8), 764–9.

Lonsdale, S. (1990) *Women and Disability*, Macmillan, London.

Lukes, S. (1974) *Power: A Radical View*, British Sociological Association, Macmillan, London.

Lyon, J. (1989) Communicative Partners: Their value in reestablishing communication with aphasic adults, in *Clinical Aphasiology Conference Proceedings* (ed T.E. Prescott), 18, College-Hill Press, San Diego, California, pp. 11–17.

Mackenzie, C., LeMay, M., Lendrem, W. *et al.* (1993) A survey of aphasia services in the United Kingdom, *European Journal of Disorders of Communication*, **28**, 43–61.

Malone, R.L. (1969) Expressed attitudes of families of aphasics, *Journal of Speech and Hearing Disorders*, **34**, 146–51.

Malone, R.L., Ptacek, P.H. and Malone, M.S. (1970) Attitudes expressed by families of aphasics, *British Journal of Disorders of Communication*, **5**(2), 174–9.

Mangan, Z. and Trewhitt, P. (1993) Breaking down the communication barriers, *College of Speech and Language Therapists Bulletin*, **498**, 12–14.

Marsh, P. and Fisher, M. (1992) *Good Intentions: Developing partnership in social services*, Joseph Rowntree Foundation, York.

Marshall, J., Pound, C., White-Thomson, M. and Pring, T. (1990) The use of picture/word matching tasks to assist word retrieval in aphasic patients, *Aphasiology*, **4**(2), March-April, 167–84.

Marshall, R.C., Tompkins, C.A. and Phillips, D.S. (1982) Improvement in treated aphasia – examination of selected prognostic factors, *Folia Phoniatrica*, **34**, 305–15.

Martin, J., Meltzer, H. and Elliot, D. (1988) *The Prevalence of Disability among Adults*, Office of Population Censuses and Surveys, HMSO, London.

Martin, J., White, A. and Meltzer, H. (1989) *Disabled Adults: Services, Transport and Employment*, Office of Population Censuses and Surveys, HMSO, London.

Maxim, J. and Bryan, K. (1993) 'Talking and listening' in *Handbook for Hospital Care Assistants* (eds L. Swiatczak and S. Benson), Hawker, London.

Maxim, J. and Bryan, K. (1995) Talking and listening, in *Handbook for Care Assistants* 4th edn (eds S. Darby and S. Benson), Hawker, London.

McLellan, L. (1991) The UK experience of rehabilitation, in *The National Concept of Rehabilitation Medicine*, Proceedings of a Conference of the Disablement Services Authority and the Royal College of Physicians, Royal College of Physicians of London, London, pp. 13–20.

Meikle, M. and Wechsler, E. (1983) Response to T R Pring 2. *British Journal of Disorders of Communication*, **18**, 77.

Meikle, M., Wechsler, E., Tupper, A. *et al.* (1979) Comparative trial of volunteer and professional treatments of dysphasia after stroke. *British Medical Journal*, **2**(6182), 87–9.

Metter, E.J. (1991) Brain–behaviour relationships in aphasia studied by Positron Emission Tomography, in *Windows on the Brain. Neuropsychology's technological frontiers* (eds R.A. Zapulla, F.F. LeFever, J. Jaeger and R. Bilder), Annals of the New York Academy of Sciences, p. 620.

Minister for Disabled People (1995) *Ending discrimination against disabled people: Summary of Government proposals*. Central Office of Information, HMSO, London.

Molteno, B. and Powell, H. (1990) A back to school approach for aphasia sufferers. *Speech Therapy in Practice*, **5**(10), March, 2.

Moore, L.F. (ed.) (1985) *Motivating Volunteers*, Vancouver Volunteer Centre, Vancouver.

Morris, J. (1991) *Pride Against Prejudice: Transforming Attitudes to Disability*, The Women's Press, London.

Morris, J. (1995) *The Power to Change: Commissioning Health and Social Services with Disabled People*, Living Options Partnership Paper No. 2, the King's Fund, London.

Mulhall, D.J. (1978) Dysphasic stroke patients and the influence of their relatives. *British Journal of Disorders of Communication*, **13**(2), 127–34.

Mykyta, L.J., Bowling, J.H., Nelson, D.A. *et al.* (1976) Caring for relatives of stroke patients. *Age and Ageing*, **5**, 87–90.

National Aphasia Association (USA) n.d. (c. 1988) (a) *Impact of aphasia on patients and family: a survey.*

National Aphasia Association (USA) n.d. (c. 1988) (b) *What is the National Aphasia Association?*

NHS Executive (1995) *Stroke*, HMSO, London.

Nickels, L. and Best, W. (1993) Therapy for naming disorders (Parts 1 and 2). Conference Paper, British Aphasiology Society Conference. Warwick University.

Nocon, A. (1994) *Collaboration in Community Care in the 1990s*, Business Education Publishers Ltd., Sunderland.

Office of Health Economics (1988) *Stroke*, Current Health Problems No. 89, Office of Health Economics, London.

Oliver, M. (1983) *Social Work with Disabled People*, Macmillan, London.

Oliver, M. (1990) *The Politics of Disablement*, Macmillan, London.

Oranen, M., Sihvonen, R., Aysto, S. *et al.* (1987) Different coping patterns in the families of aphasic people, *Aphasiology*, **1**(3), 277–81.

Overs, R.P. and Belknap, E.L. (1967) Educating stroke patient families, *Journal of Chronic Diseases*, **20**, 45–51.

Pachalska, M. (1993) The concept of holistic rehabilitation of persons with aphasia, in *Aphasia Treatment: World Perspectives* (eds A.L. Holland and M.M. Forbes), Chapman & Hall, London, pp. 145–74.

Parr, S. (1994) Coping with aphasia: conversations with 20 aphasic people, *Aphasiology*, **8**(5), 457–66.

Parr, S. (1995) Everyday reading and writing in aphasia: role change and the influence of pre-morbid literacy practice, *Aphasiology*, **9**(3) 223–38.

Parr, S. and Gilpin, S. (1995) Aphasia and disability: a research project investigating the consequences and significance of aphasia, *Speaking Up*, **36** (May), 8.

Parr, S., Pound, C. and Marshall, J. (1995) A handful of power for aphasic people, *College of Speech and Language Therapists Bulletin*, **617** (May), 8–10.

Parsons, T. (1951) *The Social System*, Routledge and Kegan Paul, London.

Paton, N. (1995) Yes, but will it change anything? *Disability Now*, December, 5.

Peach, R. (1993) Clinical intervention for aphasia in the United states of America, in *Aphasia Treatment: World Perspectives* (eds A.L. Holland and M.M. Forbes), Chapman & Hall, London, pp. 335–69.

Peterson, S.E., Fox, P.T., Posner, M., Mintun, M. and Raichle, M.E. (1988) Positron emission tomographic studies of the cortical anatomy of single-word processing, *Nature*, **331**, 585–9.

Pinker, S. (1994) *The Language Instinct*, Penguin, London.

Pound, C. (1993) Attitudes to disability: Power and the therapeutic relationship. Conference Paper, British Aphasiology Society Conference. Warwick University.

Pound, C. and Sheridan, J. (1994) Back to basics? *College of Speech and Language Therapists Bulletin*, **505** (May), 4–5.

Prime Minister's Office (1991) *The Citizen's Charter: Raising the Standard*, Cm 1599, HMSO, London.

Pring, T.R. (1983) Speech therapists and volunteers – some comments on recent investigations of their effectiveness in the treatment of aphasia. *British Journal of Disorders of Communication,* **18,** 65–73.

Pring, T.R. (1986) Evaluating the effects of speech therapy for aphasics: developing the single case methodology. *British Journal of Disorders of Communication,* **21**(1), 103–116,

Purdy, T. (1985) Using volunteers in training with communication aids, in RADAR/RNID *European Conference on Technology and Communication Impairment,* Conference Papers, Institute of Education, London.

Quinteros, B., Williams, D.R.R., White, C.A.M. *et al.* (1984) The costs of using trained and supervised volunteers as part of a speech therapy service for dysphasic patients, *British Journal of Disorders of Communication,* **19,** 205–12.

Rice, B., Paull, A. and Muller, D.J. (1987) An evaluation of a social support group for spouses of aphasic partners, *Aphasiology,* **1**(3), 247–56.

Ritchie, D. (1960, 1974) *Stroke: a diary of recovery,* Faber and Faber, London.

Robinson, R.G. and Starkstein, S.E. (1990) Current research in affective disorders following stroke, *Journal of Neuropsychiatric and Clinical Neuroscience,* **2,** 1–14.

Rolland, J. and Belin, C. (1993) The person with aphasia and the workforce, in *Living with Aphasia: Psychosocial Issues* (eds D. Lafond, R. DeGiovani, Y. Joanette *et al.*), Singular Publishing Group, Inc., San Diego, California, pp. 223–42.

Rooney, M. (1989) Will 'Working for Patients' work for us? *Speech Therapy in Practice,* **4**(7), (March), 4.

Ross, A. (1990) To encourage referrals from GPs efforts should be made to educate them about speech therapy. *Speech Therapy in Practice,* Special Supplement No. 1 (March), 4–5.

Rossiter, D. (1987) Ever decreasing circles, Conference Paper at British Aphasiology Society Conference, Newcastle upon Tyne, September 1987, unpublished.

Rossiter, D. (1989) The prevalence of disability among adults: how does communication rate? *Speech Therapy in Practice,* **5**(1) (June), 7–8.

Rossiter, D. and McInally, K. (1989) Aphasia services: provision or privation? *College of Speech Therapists Bulletin,* **499** (September), 4–6.

Royal Association for Disability and Rehabilitation (1994) *Half Measures,* Royal Association for Disability and Rehabilitation, London.

Royal College of Speech and Language Therapists Bulletin (1995a) SLT Advocacy in court, **519** (July), 1 and 3.

Royal College of Speech and Language Therapists Bulletin (1995b) SLT: Love it? Leave it?, **520** (August), 1 and 3.

Safilios-Rothschild, C. (1981) Disabled persons' self-definitions and their implications for rehabilitation, in *Handicap in a Social World* (eds A. Brechin, P. Liddiard and J. Swain), Hodder and Stoughton, Sevenoaks.

Sasanuma, S. (1993) Aphasia treatment in Japan, in *Aphasia Treatment: World Perspectives* (eds A.L. Holland and M.M. Forbes), Chapman & Hall, London, pp. 175–98.

Schwartz, M.F., Saffran, E.M. and Fink, R.B. (1994) Mapping therapy: a treatment programme for agrammatism. *Aphasiology*, **8**(1), 19–54.

Seron, X. and de Partz, M.-P. (1993) The re-education of aphasics: between theory and practice, in *Aphasia Treatment: World Perspectives* (eds A.L. Holland and M.M. Forbes), Chapman & Hall, London, pp. 131–44.

Silburn, L. (1994) Innovative Practice: A social model in a medical world: the development of the integrated living team as part of the strategy for younger physically disabled people in North Derbyshire, in *On Equal Terms: Working with Disabled People* (ed. S. French), Butterworth-Heinemann, pp. 250–6.

Slack, P. and Mulville, F. (1988) *Sweet Adeline: a journey through care*. Macmillan, Basingstoke and London.

Smith, L. (1985) Communicative activities of aphasic adults: a survey. *British Journal of Disorders of Communication*, **20**(1), 31–44.

Smith, R. (1987) *Unemployment and Health*, Oxford University Press, Oxford.

Solome, M. (1989) The Aphasia Association: Aphasics co-operate with professionals. *Aphasia European Congress*. Abstracts, Brussels.

Solomon, J. (1995) *A survey of present stroke contracts*, Royal College of Physicians, London.

Sparkes, C. (1993) The impact of language loss on marriage. *College of Speech and Language Therapists Bulletin*, **494** (June), 9–11.

Speakeasy Club (1988a) *Relatives' Handbook*, Speakeasy Club, Bury.

Speakeasy Club (1988b, 1994b) *Volunteers' Handbook*, Speakeasy Club, Bury.

Speech Therapy in Practice (1987) Survey results: use of volunteers is widespread, **2**(4), 28–9.

Spencer, C. (1994) Working with volunteers, *College of Speech and Language Therapists Bulletin*, **505** (May), 11.

Stevens, S., LeMay, M., Gravell, R. and Cook, K. (1992) *Working with Elderly People: Communication Workshops*, Far communications, Kibworth.

Stevenson, O. and Parsloe, P. (1993) *Community Care and Empowerment*, Joseph Rowntree Foundation, York.

(The) Stroke Association Community Services (1993a) *Dysphasic Support*. (Information leaflet), The Stroke Association, London.

(The) Stroke Association Community Services (1993b) *Family Support* (Information leaflet), The Stroke Association, London.

(The) Stroke Association Community Services (1993c) *Information Centres* (Information leaflet), The Stroke Association, London.

Swaffield, L. (1990) *Stroke: the Complete Guide to Recovery and Rehabilitation*. Thorsons, Wellingborough.

Swain, J., Finkelstein, V., French, S. and Oliver, M. (eds) (1993) *Disabling Barriers – Enabling Environments*, Sage, London.

Syder, D. (1989) Time to act on words. *Health Service Journal*, 26 January, pp. 106–7.

Syder, D., Body, R., Parker, M. and Boddy, M. (1993) *The Sheffield Screening Test for Acquired Language Disorders*, NFER-Nelson, Windsor.

Thompson, P., Buckle, J. and Lavery, M. (1988) *Not the OPCS Report: Being disabled costs more than they said*, Disablement Income Group, London.

Tomlinson Report (1992) *Report of the Inquiry into London's Health Service, Medical Education and Research*, HMSO, London.

Townsend, P. (1981) The structured dependency of the elderly: a creation of social policy in the twentieth century. *Ageing and Society*, **1**(1), 5–28.

Trewhitt, P. (1995) Equal opportunities and the management of long-term communication disability, *College of Speech and Language Therapists Bulletin*, **617** (May), 12–13.

Turner, P. (1989) Budget Cinderellas, *Health Service Journal*, 15 June, 734.

Twigg, J. (1989) Models of carers: how do social care agencies conceptualise their relationships with informal carers? *Journal of Social Policy*, **18**(1) (January), 53–66.

Twigg, J. and Atkin, K. (1994) *Carers Perceived: policy and practice in informal care*. Open University Press, Buckingham.

van der Gaag, A. (1993) *Audit: a manual for speech and language therapists*, College of Speech and Language Therapists, London.

Wade, D.T. (1983) Can aphasic patients with stroke do without speech therapy? *British Medical Journal*, **286**, 50.

Wade, D. and Langton Hewer, R. (1987) Epidemiology of some neurological diseases with special reference to workload on the NHS, *International Rehabilitation Medicine*, **8**, 129–37.

Wade, D.T., Langton Hewer, R., Skilbeck, C. and David, R. (1985) *Stroke: A critical approach to diagnosis, treatment and management*, Chapman & Hall Medical, London.

Währborg, P. (1991) *Assessment and Management of Emotional and Psychosocial Reactions to Brain Damage and Aphasia*, Far Communications, Kibworth.

Währborg, P. and Borenstein, P. (1989) Family therapy in families with an aphasic member. *Aphasiology*, **3**(1), 93–8.

Waine, B. (1991) *The Rhetoric of Independence*, Berg, Oxford.

Ward, M. and Waugh, E. (1983) Report of the ALBSU Special Development Project Basic Education for Dysphasic Adults. Unpublished report.

Wertz, R.T. (1989) Utilizing trained volunteers to treat aphasia, in *Clinical Aphasiology Conference Proceedings* (ed. T.E. Prescott), 18 College-Hill Press, San Diego, California, pp. 5–10.

Wertz, R.T., Weiss, D.G., Aten, J.L. *et al.* (1986) Comparison of clinic, home and deferred language treatment for aphasia. A Veterans Administration Co-operative study. *Archives of Neurology*, **43**, 653–8.

Wood, P. (1989) Conceptual issues underlying disability research. In *Researching Disability: Methodological Issues*. ESRC survey methods seminar series: report of the June 1989 seminar.

Wood, R. (1988) Disabled people point the way forward. *Social Work Today*, **21** January, 16–17.

World Health Organization (1980) *International Classification of Impairments,*

Disabilities and Handicaps. World Health Organization, Geneva.

Worrall, L. (1992) Functional communication assessment: an Australian Perspective. *Aphasiology*, **6**(1), 105–110.

Appendix A
Abbreviations

ABE	adult basic education
ADA	Action for Dysphasic Adults
AIA	Association Internationale Aphasie
ALBSU	Adult Literacy and Basic Skills Unit
BAS	British Aphasiology Society
CHSA	Chest, Heart and Stroke Association (in England and Wales this became the Stroke Association in 1991; Scotland and Northern Ireland continue to have separate CHSAs)
CSLT	College of Speech and Language Therapists (this was the College of Speech Therapists until 1991; in 1995 it became the Royal College of Speech and Language Therapists)
CST	College of Speech Therapists (see note under CSLT)
CT	computed tomography
DHA	District Health Authority
DoH	Department of Health
FHSA	Family Health Services Authority
GNVQ	General National Vocational Qualification(s)
GP	General Practitioner (family doctor)
LRT	London Regional Transport
MRI	magnetic resonance imaging
NHS	National Health Service
OPCS	Office of Population Censuses and Surveys
PACE	Promoting Aphasics' Communicative Effectiveness
PALPA	Psycholinguistic Assessments of Language Processing in Aphasia
PET	positron emission tomography
RADAR	Royal Association for Disability and Rehabilitation

RCSLT   Royal College of Speech and Language Therapists (see note under CSLT)

UK   United Kingdom (England, Wales, Scotland and Northern Ireland)

USA   United States of America

VSS   Volunteer Stroke Scheme/Service (this became Stroke Association Dysphasic Support service in 1993)

WHO   World Health Organization

WRVS   Women's Royal Voluntary Service

Appendix B
Resource list

Audiocassettes:

ADA   *Living with Dysphasia* 1993

ADA   *Personal Insights* 1995

Videocassettes:

ADA   *Say the Words that Matter*

The Stroke Association   *Back to Square One* (out of production)

Why Me? The Experience of Stroke

In Their Own Time

Play

Jean Claude van Italie   *The Traveller*
Based on the experience of theatre director Joseph Chaikim who became aphasic
following a stroke in 1983. First produced in the USA in 1986. European
premier at The Haymarket, Leicester, 1st
October 1987 with David Threlfall in the
title role.

Film

Marcel Simard   *Les Mots Perdus*
A film in four seasons (1993)
Produced by Virage, Québec, Canada

Leaflets/Booklets:

ADA   *How to Help* ... series by Jane Marshall and
Eva Carlson (1993)

1 How to *help* the dysphasic person in the *early stages*

2 How to *help* the dysphasic person with *comprehension* and *speech*

3 How to *help* the dyphasic person with *reading* and *writing*

4 How to *help* the dysphasic person with *total communication*

5 *Complicating factors* with dysphasia

Lost for Words

Stroke and dysphasia: Drawing the picture together (1990)

The *How to Help* ... series is also available in French and German. Other translations are in the offing.

When Granny Couldn't Speak by Rebecca Lisle (1996)

The Stroke Association

S2   *Learning to speak again*

S25 *Cognitive problems following stroke* by Barbara A Wilson

For Service Providers:

ADA

National Directory: National Register of Language

Opportunities for those with Dysphasia and their Families (1995)

Volume 1: Scotland and Northern Ireland

Volume 2: Northern, Yorkshire, Trent, North Western and Mersey

Volume 3: Wales, Heart of England, West Midlands, Wessex and South Western

Volume 4: East Anglia, London and South East England

Author index

Subject index

Page numbers appearing in **bold** refer to figures, page numbers appearing in *italics* refer to tables